The Massey Lectures Series

The Massey Lectures are co-sponsored by CBC Radio, House of Anansi Press, and Massey College in the University of Toronto. The series was created in honour of the Right Honourable Vincent Massey, former governor general of Canada, and was inaugurated in 1961 to provide a forum on radio where major contemporary thinkers could address important issues of our time.

This book comprises the 2005 Massey Lectures, "Race Against Time," broadcast in November 2005 as part of CBC Radio's *Ideas* series. The producer of the series was Philip Coulter; the executive producer was Bernie Lucht.

Stephen Lewis

Stephen Lewis is the United Nations Secretary-General's special envoy for HIV/AIDS in Africa, a commissioner on the World Health Organization's Commission on Social Determinants of Health, senior advisor to Columbia University's Mailman School of Public Health, and director of the Stephen Lewis Foundation (www.stephenlewisfoundation.org). He has had extensive experience as a politician, diplomat, and humanitarian, including tenures as leader of Ontario's New Democratic Party, as Canadian ambassador to the UN, as special advisor on Africa to the UN Secretary-General, and as deputy executive director of UNICEF. In particular, he is a passionate advocate for the rights and needs of children and women. Stephen Lewis is a Companion of the Order of Canada, has been awarded the Pearson Peace Medal, was named *Maclean's* magazine's inaugural "Canadian of the Year" in 2003, was listed by *TIME* magazine as one of the 100 most influential people in the world in 2005, and, amongst other awards, holds twenty-two honorary degrees from Canadian universities. He lives in Toronto, Canada.

RACE AGAINST TIME

STEPHEN LEWIS

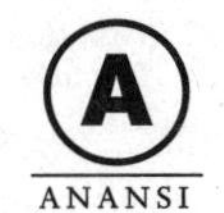

Published in 2005 by
House of Anansi Press Inc.
110 Spadina Avenue, Suite 801
Toronto, ON, M5V 2K4
Tel. 416-363-4343
Fax 416-363-1017
www.anansi.ca

Distributed in Canada by
HarperCollins Canada Ltd.
1995 Markham Road
Scarborough, ON, M1B 5M8
Toll free tel. 1-800-387-0117

Distributed in the United States by
Publishers Group West
1700 Fourth Street
Berkeley, CA 94710
Toll free tel. 1-800-788-3123

CBC and Massey College logos used with permission

House of Anansi Press is committed to protecting our natural environment. As part of our efforts, this book is printed on Rolland Enviro paper: it contains 100% post-consumer recycled fibres, is acid-free, and is processed chlorine-free.

09 08 07 06 05 3 4 5 6

LIBRARY AND ARCHIVES CANADA CATALOGUING IN PUBLICATION DATA

Lewis, Stephen, 1937–
Race against time / Stephen Lewis.

(CBC Massey lectures series)
ISBN 0-88784-733-1

1. Human rights. 2. Poverty. 3. Africa. 4. Millennium Development Goals.
I. Title. II. Series.

JC571.L534 2005 323 C2005-905162-0

Cover design: Bill Douglas at The Bang
Front-cover photographs: (top) Digital Vision;
(bottom) copyright © Tamela Hultman/allAfrica.com. All rights reserved.
Typesetting: Brian Panhuyzen

Canada Council
for the Arts

Conseil des Arts
du Canada

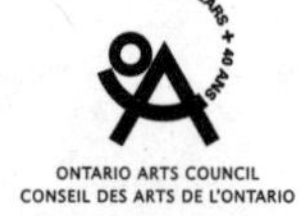

We acknowledge for their financial support of our publishing program the Canada Council for the Arts, the Ontario Arts Council, and the Government of Canada through the Book Publishing Industry Development Program (BPIDP).

Printed and bound in Canada

To the women living with AIDS in Africa
Indomitable, Resilient, Courageous
One day the world will come to its senses.

Contents

PREFACE

THIS IS NOT a *pro forma* preface. I have a number of things I want to say about the writing of these lectures.

First, I'm addicted to the spoken word; speaking is my vocation. But there is a cadence and rhythm — sometimes even feckless abandon — to a speech which doesn't always translate comfortably to the page. I readily admit that it was difficult to find a rapprochement between the spoken and the written word. These are five separate lectures, delivered in five separate cities. There will therefore be some redundancy and the occasional clunky-sounding word or phrase — the eccentricities of speaking.

Second, because the due date for the writing of the book significantly preceded the delivery of the lectures themselves, I was perpetually hostage to events. My basic theme is the Millennium Development Goals, and I found myself constantly jousting with international meetings (like the G8 Summit) whose relevance was key but whose dates fell between the book and the lectures. By breaking the deadline rules, I managed to delay the completion of the text until some of the crucial meetings had come and gone. It was a trifle sneaky, but very satisfying.

I've struggled valiantly with this swirl of ongoing events; I can only hope that the lectures are seen to have an inherent and independent integrity.

Third, inevitably I couldn't do more than scratch the surface of a number of critical issues; they'll have to remain for a future book. If there had been time or space, I would have liked to confront the frequent preoccupation with African "governance" on the one hand and African "corruption" on the other. The corruption issue is particularly gnawing since it forever seems to tarnish the continent's right to health and recovery. I always flinch when people bandy about charges of corruption: it constitutes such a double standard in the face of our own Canadian sponsorship scandal, or the billions unaccounted for in the U.S. administration of Iraq's oil revenues. I've learned that corruption is an accusation most eagerly hurled by people in glass houses.

Finally, I wrote these lectures as someone who loves the United Nations and the ideals it embodies. I'm not an apologist, but I'm certainly a devotee. The United Nations has shaped the last twenty-one years of my life, and I've cherished every job that I've held in the heartland of multilateralism. The first was my appointment — an entire surprise — as Canadian ambassador to the United Nations from 1984 to 1988, followed by positions with UNICEF (including deputy executive director), specific roles with two previous Secretaries-General, with the Economic Commission for Africa, the International Labour Organization, and the United Nations Development Fund for Women, with UNAIDS, and culminating in my present work, since 2001, as the Secretary-General's special envoy on HIV/AIDS in Africa.

In the course of the last two decades, therefore, I've watched the United Nations from the inside, and have had the privilege of working with international civil servants throughout the secretariat and in many of the major agencies. I've also had the experience (especially in the UNICEF and envoy roles) of observing the work of the UN on the ground, in-country, where its work is most evident and truly appreciated.

In the process, I've witnessed both the strengths and weaknesses of multilateralism, especially in the domains of development and humanitarian intervention. I glory in the strengths and I'm appalled by the weaknesses. As a result, these lectures are not confined to adoration; there's some heavy-duty criticism. That part of it hasn't been easy; I'm loath to reproach the United Nations.

And yet, in far too many instances I've seen wilful inertia or outright irresponsibility at work within the UN family. I know the wondrous heights the UN can scale (just think of the eradication of smallpox, or the near-eradication of polio); there's neither need nor justification to wallow in the trough of mediocrity. When it happens, it should be identified. Too much is at stake. The Secretary-General talks volubly of UN reform; if there is to be reform, then the things that are out of whack need to be identified and put right.

Everyone, every government in the international arena, is talking UN renewal. Apart from being the centrepiece of the discussions in the General Assembly in September 2005, it will remain at the top of the agenda for the foreseeable future. Inevitably, the main focus of renewal is on the Security Council, or resolutions on terrorism, or the new Human Rights Council. What I have attempted to do in these lectures is to join the debate, by providing my own view of renewal, a renewal which speaks to the development and humanitarian ethos — the side of the UN charter that is so often neglected.

This has not been an easy undertaking for me; in fact, it's been quite painful in places. It seems to me that those of us who care about the United Nations have an ethical responsibility to point out its failings and to suggest constructive alternatives. There is a tendency to think that dissent should be contained or that self-censorship is to be applauded. I regard both sentiments as the last refuge of an intellectual wimp.

On the other hand, I realize that I'm running a risk in these lectures. Some of the things I'm saying, some of the arguments I'm making, will rub UN officialdom and various politicians the wrong way. They may wish to exact retribution. I've thought a lot about that because I so value the job I've been permitted to do.

But it seems to me that the mark of a true loyalist is to be honest with those to whom he or she is loyal. So I've taken candour to heart. Unless the foibles and failings of the UN on the development and humanitarian agendas are discussed publicly, they will never change. I believe to the depths of my being that they must change, because never has humankind been in greater need of a trusted, rational, purposeful, and principled United Nations.

If this were five years ago, and I had been given the privilege of delivering the Massey Lectures, I might have adopted a more conciliatory tone. I might have subjected the Millennium Development Goals to a measured analytic discourse. But 2005 is not 2000. In the interim I've been emotionally torn asunder by the onslaught of AIDS, and it has profoundly changed my view of the world. My life is consumed by this plague. I can't deny it; it colours everything I believe and say. As I write these words, I have many African friends who are even now gasping for a few more days of life. My impatience with the United Nations and with western and African governments stems, in large part, from their dilatory — often unconscionably dilatory — response to the pandemic. While it is true that I've been tough in places in these lectures, I don't believe I've gone overboard. Indeed, as measured against the human apocalypse, the reader may even conclude that I've been restrained.

— August 2005

ACKNOWLEDGEMENTS

I COULD NOT possibly have produced these lectures without the indispensable assistance of my very good friend Paula Donovan. She read every word, scrutinized every paragraph, vetted every page, and suggested significant changes, almost all of which I have incorporated. Some of the best ideas in Chapter 5 also come from Paula, ideas which I have shamelessly filched without attribution.

I must also thank, deeply and abidingly, my wife, Michele Landsberg, my son, Avi Lewis, and my daughter-in-law, Naomi Klein, for the review of the text at various stages along the way. They were hugely encouraging at every moment when I was suffering a crisis of confidence, and they provided insight and comment galore.

For the title, I have Judy Jackson the filmmaker to thank, who first employed it as the title of a documentary about AIDS on *The Nature of Things*. I therefore must also extend my appreciation for its use to host David Suzuki and Executive Producer Michael Allder of the CBC.

I was also assisted in the editing process by David Hayes and Kevin Linder at House of Anansi Press. I am indebted to Anansi's patience, since I was slightly overdue — by about four months — in the delivery of the manuscript. And of course I offer full appreciation to the CBC and to Massey College for having extended the invitation to me to deliver the lectures.

And no thanks would be complete without acknowledgement of the help of my executive assistant and close colleague, Christina Magill. In her usual astonishingly competent fashion, with cosmic unflappability, she handled all of the particulars and problems that arose along the way.

As much as I am beholden to all of the above, any damning faults or execrable errors are purely my own.

I

CONTEXT: IT SHAMES AND DIMINISHES US ALL

I HAVE SPENT the last four years watching people die. Nothing in my adult life prepared me for the carnage of HIV/AIDS. Between 1998 and 2000, I participated in a study of the Rwandan genocide, commissioned by the Organization of African Unity. Visits to commemorative sites reminiscent of Auschwitz, encounters with survivors, interviews with women who had been raped repeatedly during the genocide — it all felt like a descent into depravity from which there was no escape. And yet, somehow, because it came to an end, because the little country of Rwanda is managing to piece itself together, step by painful step, there is at least a sense that the horrific events are rendered unto history. That is not to say that we should ever forget, only to say that it is over.

But the pandemic of HIV/AIDS feels as though it will go on forever. The adult medical wards of the urban hospitals are filled with AIDS-related illnesses, men, women, wasted and dying; aluminum coffins wheeling in and out in Kafkaesque rotation; in the pediatric wards, nurses tenderly removing the bodies of infants; funerals occupying the weekends, cemeteries running out of grave sites; in the villages, hut after hut yields a picture of a mother, usually a young woman, in the final throes of life. No one is untouched. Everyone has a heartbreaking story to tell. Virtually every country in East and southern Africa is a nation of mourners.

In July 2005, I was travelling in Kenya, visiting an association of women living with AIDS in a slum suburb of the city of Nairobi. The slum was teeming with orphans, being cared for by the women left alive. In every such instance, there's always some kind of "performance" for the visitors, as though the encounter would be incomplete or marred without it. We gathered outside one of the crumbling homes, where six children, ranging in age from five to twelve, wearing ragged green school uniforms, chanted the largely tuneless, funereal dirge of their own composition: "Here we are, the orphans, carrying our parents in their coffins to their graves." The song ended with the words "Help, Help, Help." And then there came forward a girl of ten, a translator at her side, to describe the last remnants of her mother's life. It was awful. The mother had clearly died only a few days before, and as the young girl described the journeys in and out of hospital, and her mother's final hours, she wept so uncontrollably, her words strangled in loss, the tears gushing — not falling, or streaming, or pouring, but gushing — down her cheeks and onto her sweater and then to the ground, as though in this one child, in this one moment, all the untold agony of the pandemic was incarnate.

In this context, in the midst of this nightmare, in this race against time, the Millennium Development Goals (MDGs) seem strangely miscast. And yet, the MDGs were and are the ostensible subject of these lectures. In a way which no one could have forecast, the MDGs have become the centrepiece of public policy in country after country, especially the countries of the developing world. They emerged from the UN's Millennium Assembly in 2000, when the international community, with surprising unanimity, decided that a number of targets had to be set for the year 2015, essentially to confront the eviscerating poverty of large parts of the developing world, and Africa in particular. So allow me to recapitulate the eight MDGs for you, remembering that the target date is 2015: cut the worst of poverty and hunger in half, achieve universal primary education, promote gender equality, reduce by two-thirds the under-five child mortality rate, reduce by three-quarters the maternal mortality rate, halt and reverse the spread of HIV/AIDS and malaria, ensure environmental sustainability, and develop a global partnership for development.

It is my intention, during the course of the lectures, to address, directly or indirectly, all of the goals, save that of environmental sustainability. The complexities of environmental policy, including climate change, seem to me to require an entire Massey lecture series on their own.

It is important to note at the outset, that every learned commentator, from the World Bank to the United Nations

Development Programme (UNDP) asserts that not a one of the high-prevalence HIV countries will make the goals. In fact, sub-Saharan Africa is so poor, so besieged by a range of communicable diseases, so lacking in human capacity, so barren of infrastructure, that it is entirely likely that not a single country in the region will make the goals. Nor has that situation been radically altered by the G8 Summit in July 2005.

I have to say that the ongoing plight of Africa forces me to perpetual rage. It's all so unnecessary, so crazy that hundreds of millions of people should be thus abandoned.

The easy canard of course is to say that Africa is a basket-case of anti-democratic chaos. The detractors finger eastern Congo, northern Uganda, Sudan, and Zimbabwe as examples of countries in such turmoil as to defy democratic development. And of course, in large measure, in those specific instances, the detractors are right. But there are fifty-three countries in sub-Saharan Africa, increasing numbers of them embracing democracy, and it's the height of arrogance to consign them all to some self-inflicted purgatory.

It's important to remember that Africa was left in dreadful shape by the departing colonial powers, and was subsequently whip-sawed between ideological factions in the Cold War. But rather more decisive, it was also delivered to the depredations of the so-called IFIs — the collection of International Financial Institutions dominated by the World Bank and the International Monetary Fund (colloquially known as "the Bank" and "the Fund"), and including the African Development Bank and other regional development banks. The result of the IFIs' destructive power over Africa was to compromise the social sectors, particularly the health and education sectors of the continent to this day.

History conveniently overlooks the policies of the Bank and the Fund. I don't intend to. In the late eighties and nineties, the IFIs launched what are famously known as Structural Adjustment Programs (SAPs). Stripped of the econometric gobbledegook and overblown ideological formulations, SAPs were Reaganomics gone berserk. It is my contention that for almost twenty years, those rigid fundamentalist policies did extraordinary damage to African economies from which they have yet to recover.

Everyone understood that SAPs were driven by "conditionality." The Bank and the Fund would offer loans in return for which the recipient countries would have to live with certain conditions. The conditions ranged from the sale of public sector corporations, to the imposition of "cost-sharing" (the euphemism for user fees imposed on health and education), to savage cut-backs in employment levels in the public service, mostly in the social sectors. To this day, the cut-backs haunt Africa: the IFIs continue to impose "macroeconomic" limits on the numbers of people (think nurses and teachers) who can be hired, and if that doesn't do the trick, there are financial limits placed on the amount of money that can be spent on the social sectors as a percentage of a country's gross national product (GNP). The damage is dreadful. One of the critical reasons for Africa's inability to respond adequately to the pandemic can be explained by user fees in health care (i.e., people can't afford to pay for treatment) and user fees in education (i.e., school fees, which helps to explain why so many orphans are out of school). Simply put, at the heart of structural adjustment policies there lay two absolutes: Curtail and decimate the public sector; enhance, at any cost, the private sector. There was a lot of additional palaver about exchange rates and export policy, but those nostrums had only minimal influence on economies that were barely functioning.

I want to share with you a little of the background of all of this because, almost accidentally, I was somewhat involved.

Back in 1986, the United Nations did something it had never before done in its history: it held a Special Session on one region of the world, and that region was Africa. It's worth noting that Africa was even then considered the most beleaguered continent in the world, and that was before HIV/AIDS burst full-blown on the scene. The Special Session lasted a full week, and it was decided in advance that a western country would serve as chair of the session, the chair to be chosen from the western country group (known, if you can believe it, as WEOG, Western Europe and Others Group). Canada kindly put my name forward, and because it's positively uncouth, within the group itself, to challenge another country's yearnings, I was given that privileged post.

It was the toughest role I undertook in my four years at the United Nations. The Cold War was still raging, and the eastern bloc, led by the then Soviet Union and East Germany were bloody-minded in the extreme. Every clause of our intended final document was debated in an atmosphere of polarized frenzy, and I suppose it's fair to say that the United States was only slightly less volatile than the Soviet consortium. Along the way, the acrimonious debate nearly went off the rails on several occasions, the most dramatic of which occurred right at the last moment, and serves to illustrate just how nutty and capricious the world of diplomacy can be.

It was 4:00 in the morning of June 1, 1986, in Conference Room 2 of the UN building in New York. All 159 countries were in attendance. The place was packed. I triumphantly gavelled the meeting to silence and announced that we had reached a consensus; we had an agreed document. The room broke into loud, prolonged applause until it was noticed that the delegate from Senegal was requesting the floor. The delegate occupying Senegal's seat was the then foreign minister, Ibrahim Fall, and Senegal itself was the "chair" of the African group, appointed to speak on behalf of the group as a whole.

"We do not have agreement, Mr. President" (in the deliciously inflated vocabulary of the United Nations, "chairpersons" are "presidents"). I was completely taken aback. "How can you say that, Mr. Minister? We've passed every clause after full debate!" He replied, "Mr. President, the word 'colonialism' does not appear in the document, and until it does, we have no consensus."

There then ensued a minor socio-drama of such unbridled diplomatic absurdity as to remind one of Ionesco. I announced a fifteen-minute adjournment. I called the Senegalese foreign minister to a little secretariat office at the back of the conference room (he was a good friend, by the way) and asked him what the devil he was up to. He repeated his insistence that there was no agreement until the word "colonialism" appeared in the text, and assured me that he was speaking on behalf of the entire African group. I reminded him that I was a good friend of the African group, and expressed the view that surely he wouldn't jeopardize a landmark agreement for the sake of one word. He laughed and said that was exactly what he was saying, and I'd better find an answer or the meeting would collapse in disarray.

I told him to hang on, and then sought out the two key western ambassadors from France and the United Kingdom. The French ambassador was an amiable patrician who had to be consulted because he was, well, the French ambassador. The British ambassador, one Sir John Thomson, was a thoroughly cultivated and decent chap who recognized just how serious things were, but didn't know the answer to the conundrum, and felt personally compromised because the more senior ministerial members of his delegation had either returned to London or gone to bed. I said, "John, you've got to find a way out of this." He pondered for a while and said that the only additional wording he could think of was to say something like, "The problems of Africa are explained, in part, by colonialism, and in part, by the failings of the African leadership itself." I said, "Come on, John, they're not going to be able to accept that." He replied that it was the best he could do, and I should at least give it a shot by taking it back to the Senegalese minister.

I did. I read Minister Fall the proposed wording. He smiled, and said, "That's fine. We have agreement." I looked at him dumbfounded, and asked how he could possibly accept wording so incriminating of African leadership. He said, simply, "It has the word 'colonialism.'" I must admit, I started to laugh, and said, endearingly, "You son-of-a-bitch, you don't care what the context is, so long as you have your precious word?" "That's right," he smiled, again. (In the upshot, the final phrasing was slightly different, but "colonialism" was firmly embedded in the text in all its glory.)

Thus it was that a supposedly resurgent Africa finally emerged at 5:00 in the morning of June 1, 1986. The room started to cheer for a second time. Little did we know what was coming.

The basic rationale for the unanimous agreement was to have Africa improve its governance (you will recall that at that point in history, there were a number of despots running African countries who had taken power by force), in return for which the donors would ensure that resources flowed to the continent. Many countries of Africa made a determined effort to honour their side of the bargain; the donors, specifically working through the Bank and the Fund, unleashed structural adjustment.

It was immediately evident that the Bank policies would do severe damage. Both the Bank and the Fund were treating Africa as though it consisted of mature economies to whom western economic protocols would apply. The upper echelons of the Bank and the Fund talked the worldly language of "macroeconomic adjustment," while Africa shredded its social sectors, and poverty intensified. In fact, the constant increase in levels of poverty should have sounded a high-decibel alarm; instead the cerebral aristocrats of the IFIs ploughed ahead as if financial architecture mattered far more than human vulnerability.

I watched the growing controversy over policy first-hand. I was permitted to do so because of a decision made by the office of the Secretary-General which, because of the way it happened, prompts me to yet another discursive aside. You will have to forgive me for these occasional detours during the course of the lectures: they illumine the curious way in which the United Nations works, and on those grounds may be interesting.

In this instance, during the month of August 1986, as a direct result of the Special Session, I was called by the director general of the Department of International Economic Co-operation, Mr. Jean Ripert (known affectionately as "Beyond Repair"), and asked whether I'd like to serve as the Secretary-General's representative for Africa. I jumped at the chance and immediately said yes. Several weeks passed before I heard anything more, and then I was summoned to the thirty-eighth floor of the secretariat building (the celestial climes of the office of the Secretary-General), and met with one of his most senior officials (who shall remain nameless).

As expected, he raised the question of the Africa representative, and I confirmed my eager interest. He then said — I remember the words exactly — "How much do you want?" I was utterly confused; I simply didn't understand. He repeated the question, this time with particular accent on the word "much." It suddenly came to me — forgive the naïveté — that he was talking about money. I was incredulous. I explained that I already had a job, I was the Canadian ambassador, and I was well remunerated. He looked at me curiously and said, "You mean you don't want to be paid?" I explained again that not only did I not want to be paid, but it would constitute both double-dipping and a probable conflict of interest. His face shone with cascading relief, he vigorously shook my hand, and it all ended in a hug.

I left the office wondering to myself just how much money the United Nations paid out in similar circumstance.

Because of the formal appointment as the Secretary-General's representative, I was privy to a fascinating series of events meant to follow up on the Special Session.

Here's how it played itself out. Immediately after the Special Session, the United Nations established the Inter-Agency Task Force on Africa, specifically created to oversee the implementation of the consensus document. The task force met every couple of months, in places as disparate as Khartoum and Geneva, and the attendance was always surprisingly good; virtually every UN agency, including the Bank and the IMF, although the IMF didn't deign to turn up as often as the others.

The Task Force almost immediately split into three factions. The first comprised the coterie from the IFIs in attendance at any given meeting. At the very least, the Bank's vice-president for Africa was present, accompanied by the chief economist, and occasionally someone from the Fund. Then there was the other end of the spectrum: the chair of the Inter-Agency Task Force was Professor Adebayo Adedeji, executive secretary of the Economic Commission for Africa, based in Addis Ababa. "Prof," as he was everywhere known, was one of the most knowledgeable African leaders I have ever encountered. His vice-chair was Richard Jolly (now Sir Richard Jolly), deputy-executive director of UNICEF, and a man universally admired for a truly astonishing intellectual blend of brilliance and decency. The secretary was Sadig Rashid, Adedeji's right arm at the Economic Commission for Africa, prodigiously informed and prodigiously hard-working. And I was part of that little group as a member of the Task Force ex officio. By far the greatest number of participants, representing a range of UN agencies, were in the middle somewhere although, in every crucial vote, they sided with the Adedeji–Jolly alliance.

The battles and bitterness knew no bounds. The World Bank representative, attired in a double-breasted blue serge suit, was clearly unamused by the entire process. Why in the world should the World Bank check in with any group of mortals so palpably of lesser grasp? And why should the Bank suffer the indignity of explanation? It's hard to convey the harshness of the words that were exchanged. We loathed each other, and from Professor Adedeji and Richard Jolly — albeit cloaked in academic dignity — there came ever more vigorous attacks on SAPS.

Richard Jolly had written a major and memorable book called *Adjustment with a Human Face*, his effort to soften the blows inflicted by perverse economic policies. And Professor Adedeji, in a last mighty effort to derail the structural adjustment juggernaut, wrote an alternative program, designed to strengthen rather than to shred the social sectors. He countered the rigid ideological dogma of the Bank with a thoughtful, persuasive exposition of alternatives.

That initiative led to the *reductio ad absurdum* of the entire process, demonstrating just how massive was the gulf between the Bank and everyone else. Adedeji wrote his alternative strategy to be presented to an African finance minister's meeting, hosted by the Bank in Blantyre, Malawi, in 1990. Believe it or not — and it is almost beyond belief — the World Bank literally sequestered the documents upon arrival, and prevented their circulation. I'm not sure that's ever happened before in the annals of the UN!

The thing about structural adjustment is how wrong-headed the policies were and how even the apologists for the Bank gradually retreated in the face of the evidence. At one of our Inter-Agency meetings in Khartoum, attended by the Bank representatives, we passed a Khartoum Declaration in which it was said that SAPs were " rending the fabric of African society." I vividly remember a meeting on African economic recovery, held in one of the committee rooms of the UN, when I asked Mark Malloch Brown, then a vice-president of the Bank, and explicitly not an ideologue, what he felt about the lingering damage of SAPs.

His answer lives with me to this day: "Structural adjustment is dead." Malloch Brown went on to become administrator of the UNDP, and is now chief of staff to Kofi Annan; he's a remarkably gifted man, I take his words seriously.

But the truth is that structural adjustment is not dead: it's just morphed into other forms. The imposition of conditionality is still alive and well, fashioned now more often by the IMF as it continues to impose macroeconomic frameworks on impoverished African countries. I have come to the conclusion, as I travel, that the IMF simply doesn't understand the combined ravages of HIV/AIDS and poverty; simply fails to understand that you can't deny the hiring of health professionals, in the face of an apocalypse, just because you adhere religiously to some rabid economic dialectic which says that no matter how grievous the circumstance, you can't breach the macroeconomic environment. I saw it in Zambia and I saw it in Malawi, and in each case the governments were frantic, but the IMF wouldn't budge.

I remember being in Malawi in 2002 at a roundtable discussion with the vice-president and a number of civil servants from the Ministry of Finance. They were complaining bitterly about the limits imposed by the IMF on Malawi's public sector pay levels and hiring intentions. It was surreal: here you had a country with huge human capacity problems that wanted desperately to retain its professionals in health and education, and increase their numbers, but the IMF wouldn't allow them to do so. We're talking about a sovereign government, fighting the worst plague in history, with but a handful of professionals: according to the minister of health, Malawi has one-third of the nurses it needs (four thousand instead of the necessary twelve thousand) and perhaps 10 percent of the doctors (three hundred rather than three thousand) for a population of twelve million. And they weren't being allowed — I repeat, this sovereign government wasn't being allowed — to hire more staff and pay better salaries, because it would breach the macroeconomic straitjacket.

As I was leaving Malawi, I held a press conference and explicitly criticized the IMF for what I felt were wrong-headed policies. Sure enough, within a few days I received a formal letter (copy to my boss Kofi Annan) from the African director of the IMF pointing out, amongst other things, that the IMF was a member of the UN family, and the Secretary-General himself had decreed that one member of the family should not attack another in public. Talk about raising "chutzpah" to new levels. The IMF, which could barely bring itself to attend meetings of the UN agencies at country level, was suddenly a member of the "family."

Lest it cause concern amongst those of you of compassionate heart, I replied pretty strongly, making the point, which I truly believe, that the IMF just has no adequate sense of the struggle for survival in so many countries over which it holds sway. I didn't hear back. And there was no admonition from the Secretary-General.

It's interesting to see just a couple of years later how far the world has come. As recently as March 2005, the U.K. secretary of state for international development, Hilary Benn, published a new monograph titled "Partnerships for Poverty Reduction: Rethinking Conditionality" — I shall elaborate on this document in a future lecture. It amounts to a rejection of the categorical assumptions which have driven the IFIs over the course of the years. Almost simultaneously, Prime Minister Tony Blair released his massive Commission for Africa report, and criticized the World Bank and International Monetary Fund policies in words and argument rarely seen before in an establishment government document. And as if that wasn't enough, Jeffrey Sachs published in April 2005 his remarkable new book, *The End of Poverty*, in which, taking no intellectual prisoners, he excoriates the destructive policies of the Bank and the Fund. The message is clear: terrible mistakes were made in dealing with Africa.

What makes me nearly apoplectic — and I very much want to say this — is that the Bank and the Fund were fully told about their mistakes even as the mistakes were being made. It's so enraging that they refused to listen. They were so smug, so all-knowing, so incredibly arrogant, so wrong. They simply didn't respond to arguments which begged them to review the human consequences of their policies. The fact that poverty became increasingly entrenched, or that economies were not responding to the dogma as the dogma predicted, made no difference. It was a form of capitalist Stalinism. The credo was everything; the people were a laboratory.

What makes all of this so important is the need for radically new policies if Africans are to be given the opportunity to rescue their continent. The achievement of the MDGS has become a pipe dream in the minds of many because, in the five years since they were promulgated, we have learned that HIV/AIDS has sabotaged all of the socio-economic indices, and the continued damaging western policies in trade and aid and debt, serve to drive the nails into the coffins. In the bizarre circumstances of the pandemic, nails and coffins aren't just metaphors.

Take trade. There is absolutely no guarantee that the Doha round, presently in intense (if so far futile) negotiation, will be successful. Doha is the capital of the Gulf state, Qatar, where the most recent round of international trade talks was launched by the World Trade Organization (WTO) in November 2001. It's nearly four years later, and we've made glacial progress. The outstanding items are legion, ranging from intellectual property rights as they are tied to pharmaceuticals, right through to western agricultural subsidies, which most analysts seem to agree are destroying economic growth in Africa. As things now stand, there's simply no way for Africa profitably to export its own primary agricultural commodities.

The resolution of trade inequities cannot be met by the G8, as the summit in Gleneagles definitively confirmed. It can only be met by the meeting of the WTO in December 2005. But there seems little likelihood that the distorting trade subsidies will be abandoned. At present, the European Union and the United States together subsidize their farmers to the tune of $350 billion (U.S.

dollars) a year; it equals five times the amount that is ploughed into foreign aid. If I may offer an evocative juxtaposition: Every cow in the European Union is subsidized to the tune of two dollars a day, while between four hundred and five hundred million Africans live on less than a dollar a day.

There is, alas, no relief in sight. In fact, if anything, the prospects for relief have declined. The rifts within the European Union are increasingly pronounced, and the electoral loss in North Rhine-Westphalia of the ruling party in Germany, combined with France's bitter defeat in the vote on the European constitution, suggests that neither country will want a battle with its farmers.

But that doesn't stop the siren sounds of mollification. Time and again, the developing countries are told that if we can just get through the Doha round, everyone will benefit, Africa in particular. Poppycock!

How well I remember the previous "Uruguay round," as it was known, negotiated through the 1980s. In fact, I have one particularly vivid recollection.

It was 1988, my term as Canada's UN representative rapidly coming to end, when I received an invitation from Maurice Strong to attend a special luncheon to discuss the state of the trade negotiations. Maurice Strong, as you know, is the famous Canadian environmentalist who has had a most distinguished international career, serving several Secretaries-General, as well as acting as a senior advisor to the World Bank, amongst a proliferation of similar portfolios. In fact Maurice is the ultimate ubiquitous internationalist.

On this occasion, he invited a cross-section of UN ambassadors to lunch to meet with his special guest, Michel Camdessus, then managing director of the International Monetary Fund. Camdessus is a learned and charming man, but I have to say that I've seldom heard such an accomplished dissertation of disingenuous claptrap. Or perhaps that's way too harsh; perhaps Camdessus really believed the line he took. If that's the case, pity the IFIs.

Mr. Camdessus argued, over a delectable *tarte au poire*, that the Uruguay round would usher in a veritable trading panacea for the developing world, and he hoped the assembled ambassadors would take that word back to their respective capitals. He spoke with such certitude, such singular authority, that I expected applause rather than discussion.

I was wrong. The developing country ambassadors were having none of it, and they took Camdessus on frontally. I remember especially my colleagues from Ghana and Singapore, heaping skepticism on Camdessus's words. They were just too smart to be led down the garden path. The Ghanaian was Victor Gbeho, later to become his country's foreign minister, and the Singaporean was Kishore Mahbubani, a formidable mind, later to repeat as his country's ambassador to the UN, and to serve as the most senior civil servant in the Singapore bureaucracy. Camdessus had bitten off more than he could chew. Gbeho and Mahbubani argued, quite simply, that there was nowhere near the political will necessary to negotiate a fair agreement, and whatever was ultimately resolved, it wouldn't help the least developed countries, most of whom are in Africa.

They were of course right. Incredibly enough, during the years under the Uruguay round, African trade actually declined from 3 percent to 1 percent of global trade! That's quite a feat in an era where trade is seen as the emancipating force for the world, the chief component, as it were, in the liberating thrust of globalization.

While the story on trade is lamentable, the story on debt is worse still. And it's a story which stretches over decades, whatever the transient sense of euphoria that emanated from Gleneagles.

For almost as long as I can remember, certainly twenty years back to the Special Session on Africa, the international community has been discussing the reduction or cancellation of African debt. There are few issues about which Africans feel more strongly. I recall the inaugural meeting of the African Development Forum, in Addis Ababa, December 2000, dedicated to HIV/AIDS. Debrework Zewdie, herself an Ethiopian of celebrated standing, then leader of the team responsible for the World Bank Multi-country HIV/AIDS Program (MAP) for Africa, explained to the thousand attendees the Bank's new programs to fight AIDS in Africa, and the fact that initial agreements had been signed with Kenya and Ethiopia. Zewdie is a force to be reckoned with, but when it turned out that the monies were in the form of loans, not grants, even though the loans carried the smallest of interest rates, the audience erupted into raucous catcalls and heckling. I could scarce credit it. It became clear that the Africans in attendance, from over thirty countries, were not prepared to pay a penny's interest on monies slated to confront the worst communicable disease in history. Quite simply, the thought of any additional debt accumulation, for any purpose, was anathema.

Zewdie, never one to be intimidated, and ever a loyalist, refused to budge. It was typical of the Bank. I remember meeting Debrework in a hallway after the session, and saying to her that I thought the policy was wrong, and she rounded on me with savage eloquence, insisting that it was I who was wrong, and in any event, it was none of my business.

Later on, however, when I had moved to the envoy role, I made it my business. I remember the circumstance clearly. It was in 2002, in the absurdly luxurious surroundings of the Sheraton Hotel executive lounge in Addis, at a meeting with Callisto Madavo, one of the two vice-presidents of the Bank for Africa. I didn't have to lay out the case for grants as opposed to loans. He quite sheepishly conceded that Bank policy had been under tremendous pressure, and that he, for one, was fighting valiantly for grants at least where HIV was concerned. His views prevailed (and by the way, I feel certain that they were also the privately held views of Debrework). Shortly after, grants trumped loans.

Throughout the 1980s and 1990s, the question of African debt was a subject of perpetual debate in international forums. It was clear to everyone that many individual African countries were spending more money on servicing the debt, both bilateral and multilateral, than those same countries were spending on health, or on education, or on health and education combined.

For two decades, at every meeting of the G8 Summit attended by heads of government, at every meeting of the G7 finance ministers, at the spring and fall meetings of the IFIs, at meetings of the London Club (an assembly of commercial banks), at every meeting of the Paris Club (those gentlemanly gatherings where the assembled senior public servants from nineteen countries celebrated international financial dogma and, in my view, showed not a tinker's damn for the human predicament), ranging over twenty years, they couldn't collectively resolve the conundrum of African debt.

It may seem hard to believe, but between 1970 and 2002, Africa acquired $294 billion of debt. Much of the debt was assumed by military dictators who profited beyond the dreams of avarice, and left for the people of their countries, the crushing burden of payment.

Over the same period, it paid back $260 billion mostly in interest. At the end of it all, Africa continued to owe upwards of $230 billion in debt. Surely that is the definition of international economic obscenity. Here you have the poorest continent in the world paying off its debt, again and again, and forever being grotesquely in hock.

Now, in an orgy of self-congratulation at the recent G8 Summit, the debt was finally seen to have been confronted. Over time, much of the bilateral debt had been cancelled, but the multilateral debt, that is, the debt owed to the World Bank, the International Monetary Fund, and the African Development Bank, continued to plague the treasuries of African countries. So when the finance ministers of the G8 met just prior to their heads of government and announced, in June 2005, that they were rescinding the debt owed to the IFIs by eighteen developing countries, most of them in Africa, hosannas soared forth. The wonderful hordes of Jubilee 2000 activists, who had tenaciously and indomitably fought the good fight on debt, felt that they had finally prevailed.

And to some degree they had. But it's purely a matter of degree. The G8 leaders, as everyone knows, confirmed the write-off of $40 billion in debt for the eighteen countries at their own summit meeting in July 2005, but the actual savings for Africa, on debt service payments annually, is roughly $1 billion. I don't diminish the amount for a moment, and I have no doubt that it will be put to good use — the government of Zambia has already announced that it will use part of the savings for the purchase of antiretroviral drugs for AIDS and for the purchase of the newest drugs to combat malaria. But please remember that this is only a start, and the hosannas should, at best, be muted in tone.

The $40 billion written off in July 2005 still leaves Africa with over $200 billion shackling its future. There are unseemly comparisons to be made. If it's Iraq, and the United States decides the debt should be cancelled, then with a snap of the Pentagon's fingers, as a peremptory order to the members of the Paris Club, 80 percent, or $31 billion, is written off overnight.

Africa never receives such treatment. I want to emphasize, I must emphasize, the damage that has been done over the years. It's great to cheer now, but what about the terrible harm that was inflicted, for more than a quarter century, by virtually enslaving whole countries to the bondage of debt? You think I exaggerate? Let me quote to you from the annual UNICEF "State of the World's Children" report of 1989 where, in one of the most eloquent and persuasive pieces of writing on debt, UNICEF, frantic at the destruction of the lives of children, decided to put on paper, whatever the risk, what they truly felt. The executive director of the time was James Grant. The incomparably talented writer, who wrote every annual report for a decade, was Peter Adamson. Here is the quote:

> Three years ago, former Tanzanian President Julius Nyerere asked the question "Must we starve our children to pay our debts?" That question has now been answered in practice. And the answer has been "Yes." In those three years, hundreds of thousands of the developing world's children have given their lives to pay their countries' debts, and many millions more are still paying the interest with their malnourished minds and bodies . . .
>
> The fact that so much of today's staggering debt was irresponsibly lent and irresponsibly borrowed would matter less if the consequences of such folly were falling on its perpetrators. Yet now, when the party is over and the bills are coming in, it is the *poor* who are being asked to pay.
>
> Today, the heaviest burden of a decade of frenzied borrowing is falling not on the military or on those with foreign bank accounts or on those who conceived the years

> of waste, but on the poor who are having to do without necessities . . . on the women who do not have enough food to maintain their health, on the infants whose minds and bodies are not growing properly . . . and on the children who are being denied their only opportunity ever to go to school.
>
> In short, it is hardly too brutal an oversimplification to say that the rich got the loans and the poor got the debts.
>
> And when the impact becomes visible in rising death rates among children . . . then it is essential to strip away the niceties of economic parlance and say that what has happened is simply an outrage against a large section of humanity. The developing world's debt, both in the manner in which it was incurred and in the manner in which it is being "adjusted to," is an economic stain on the second half of the twentieth century. Allowing world economic problems to be taken out on the growing minds and bodies of young children is the antithesis of all civilized behaviour. Nothing can justify it. And it shames and diminishes us all.

Talk about a *cri de coeur*. But I beg you especially to remember it when the politicians of today crow about their limited, sometimes even paltry accomplishments. The quote from UNICEF was talking of the 1980s. It got worse in the 1990s. Nothing we have done so far to this point begins to compensate for the harm, the sheer wickedness of yesteryear.

The fulcrum on which a different future rests is foreign aid, or Official Development Assistance (ODA) as it's known. And here the signs are truly ambiguous. It's time for me to address the G8 Summit, held at Gleneagles, Scotland, in July 2005.

To hear it from crusader Bob Geldof, the summit was a spectacular success, the greatest single gathering on behalf of Africa in the history of humankind. I'm not sure that I've captured his full addiction to hyperbole, but at least it's a nice approximation. The problem for Geldof lay in his incestuous proximity to government; as a result of his membership on the Blair Commission, and his remarkable success with the Live 8 concerts, he became an inescapable member of the Blair team, a cheerleader for the G8. It's not an unusual process, this exercise in self-hypnosis; you get caught up in the sense of power and excitement and influence, and lose perspective. But in this instance, there's too much at stake to submit to the blandishments of rock stars, whatever their celebrity status.

The simple reality is straightforward; let me set the context. It is Official Development Assistance that will tell the tale for Africa. It is Official Development Assistance that goes to the social sectors, health and education in particular, giving governments the chance, the opportunity, the hope of overcoming poverty and the burden of disease. There is no other source of funds that goes so directly to the sectors on which the most vulnerable citizens of Africa depend.

By any calculation, the G8 Summit falls short. It makes some demonstrable progress, but it will not turn Africa around. The claims of Prime Minister Blair and his G8 partners must be examined more carefully.

They must be examined against the target which Tony Blair himself embraces — the target of 0.7 percent. Canadian audiences surely recognize that it was our own Lester Pearson, in 1969, when he was foreign minister, who negotiated with other western governments the benchmark of 0.7 percent of GNP as the legitimate level of foreign aid for all industrial countries. With embarrassing irony, it needs be said that not a single one of the G7 countries has ever come close to the target, Canada included. Five countries have reached or surpassed it: Sweden, Norway, Denmark, Holland, and Luxembourg. It can legitimately be asked, why these countries, with lesser economies, and not the rich countries, with buoyant economies?

Within that 0.7 percent target, Tony Blair asked for a doubling of aid to Africa by 2010: Africa receives $25 billion now, he wants $50 billion by that date. He won't get it. The United States and Japan (the two potentially largest donors by far) don't come close to approximating the need; the promises of Germany and Italy are suspect; Canada could do much more and won't; only the United Kingdom and France have reputable credentials.

A careful parsing of G8 promises would find this portion of my lecture collapsing under the weight of numbers. So I'm going to make a catalogue of statements, and ask you to trust that I can summon the arithmetic justification.

Russia, as the non-donor member of the G8, is not included. Of the remaining G8 countries, both the United Kingdom and France have said they will deliver on the 0.7 percent target, the U.K. by 2013, France by 2012. I believe them. When they say they'll double aid to Africa by 2010, they'll double aid to Africa.

Germany and Italy are in a different category. They both bridled at reaching the European Union target for 2010, and then added the ominous caveat that whatever they contributed would be dependent on the state of their economies at the time. Moreover, Italy is, alas, frequently unreliable when it comes to matching dollars with commitments by the dates specified.

Then there's Japan. In this instance, the cascade of promises occurred right at the eleventh hour of the summit, and was heralded by Tony Blair as the breakthrough. Forgive me, but it's just not credible. Japan made four specific promises, amongst them the doubling of aid to Africa over the next three years. Japan's record on foreign aid is so abysmal (they stand at 0.18 percent of GNP, other than the United States, the lowest of all industrial nations), that it's hard to credit such a turnaround. Doubling of aid over the next three years sounds terrific until you examine the financial data. According to definitive western statistics, Japan contributed 17.7 percent of its net foreign aid to Africa in 2002/2003, a lower percentage than any other industrial country on the planet except for Austria and Greece! The amount works out to $1.5 billion dollars. Doubling it means another $1.5 billion out of the total $25 billion demanded by Blair: that's 6 percent from the second richest donor. Not even Einstein could rescue that equation.

And I'm not sure we're guaranteed the $1.5 billion. If I may be allowed a bracing dose of cynicism, it's necessary to point out that Japan wanted a seat on the Security Council, and needed the votes of the African bloc. Nothing concentrates the mind (and the treasury) more wonderfully than the quest for Security Council membership. Nothing unconcentrates the mind more rapidly than winning the seat. It's called before and after; it's often not a pretty picture.

And the picture is framed no more aesthetically by the United States. Let me state the obvious truth: If the U.S. is not onside in the Herculean effort to assist Africa, it just won't happen. I regret to say that thus far, the U.S. is a notable recalcitrant. Let me do a quick calculation, similar to that of Japan, to demonstrate the problem. It's back to Blair's target of $50 billion annually for Africa by 2010. We know that requires the doubling of current levels of ODA. The U.S. is currently providing roughly $3 billion a year; President Bush says he will indeed double it to $6 billion. But of the total $50 billion, the U.S. should be contributing $16 billion. The shortfall is therefore $10 billion. No one knows how the difference will be found.

The president touts the Millennium Challenge Account as the answer. This is a new pot of money announced by the U.S. in Monterrey in 2002, at the international conference on financing for development. It was supposed to yield several billions of dollars, increasing year by year, eventually reaching $5 billion. It hasn't happened; it hasn't come close. Rather than upping its allocation each year, Congress keeps cutting the amount. Why? Because it continually finds that, for whatever reason, the money it has already approved hasn't yet been disbursed. As of this writing, roughly 10 to 15 percent has been allocated (not yet disbursed) to four countries, only one of which is African.

And there's yet another dimension of the foreign aid saga that must be raised, if only because it's so rarely acknowledged. The truth is that every ODA figure is overstated, and I say that because so much of the money never gets to the recipient. ActionAid, the excellent U.K. development non-governmental organization (NGO), released a revealing study of G8 foreign aid on the eve of the summit. It got little coverage abroad because it disputed the received wisdom of the Blairites, but it was a fine piece of detailed analysis.

ActionAid argued — and the argument seemed to be unanswerable — that over 60 percent of ODA should be called "phantom aid," aid that is never really available for the purposes pretended. Where, then, does the money go? To "technical assistance" (otherwise known as overpriced consultants); to "tied aid" (otherwise known as the purchase of goods and services from the donor country's own firms); and to "administrative costs" (otherwise known as inflated overhead). Furthermore, according to ActionAid, and again unanswerable, is evidence that a considerable chunk of ODA comes with very particular strings attached — strings knotted by IMF conditionality, especially support for privatization. So, for instance, in the case of the groundnut industry in Senegal, or cotton marketing in Burundi and Madagascar, or urban water in Tanzania, foreign aid is available if the government will agree to privatize the industries. The conditions can be terribly damaging: in the case of Tanzania, after the U.K. Department of International Development paid the Adam Smith Institute half a million pounds to "advise" the government of Tanzania (half a million pounds which they counted as "foreign aid"), the government concluded on its own that it had to cancel the contract with a private company serving Dar es Salaam, because the poor simply couldn't afford to purchase the water.

If only 40 percent of foreign aid is "real" aid, as opposed to the phantom variety, then the G8 countries have to go well beyond doubling or tripling their pledges. Economist Jeffrey Sachs has authoritatively pointed out that of the $3 billion the U.S. annually pledges to Africa, less than $1 billion actually finds its way to poverty reduction. It becomes evident that if the phantom aid were made real, the money then available could be used to dramatic and sterling effect.

I'm weary beyond the definition of weariness at the way in which the G8 plays with figures. So far, they've had an unblemished record of betraying their promises. I do not believe that record was broken at the Gleneagles summit, except in the exotic mind of Bob Geldof. Yes, there will be more money by 2010. Yes, every penny makes a difference to Africa, and potentially, to lives saved. I'm not so foolish or curmudgeonly as to deny that reality. But spare me the claims of breakthrough. A fair trade regimen is a will-o'-the-wisp. Cancellation of debt is a fragment. The increase in foreign aid is purely conjectural. We have Kilimanjaro to climb before we meet the needs of Africa.

Unless there is a specific year-by-year timetable, with a tough reporting procedure that the whole world can measure, countries will be delinquent. What's more — and this seems to have been casually overlooked — President Bush will not be around in 2010, nor will Prime Minister Blair. President Chirac, Chancellor Schroeder, and Prime Minister Berlusconi are almost certain to be gone; in the case of Japan, it's anyone's guess whether Prime Minister Koizumi will still be around, and Prime Minister Paul Martin, too, could fade into the nether distance. These were the men who signed the document: will their successors feel bound? Don't count on it; it's too far down the road.

And then, finally, there's our own country, Canada. Here, for me, the situation is inexplicable. I have heard what the prime minister of Canada has said, and he has been good enough to talk with me directly about it. The arguments of financial incapacity are simply not persuasive.

We promised and continue to promise to reach the 0.7 percent. We are the author of the promise. Everyone knows that. Everyone on the international scene thinks it's the height of hypocrisy to propound the policy and then fail to meet it. It's no accident that all of the major witnesses who have come before the Foreign Affairs committee of the Canadian House of Commons since April 2003, from Professor Jeffrey Sachs to James Wolfensohn, just before he retired as president of the World Bank, to Richard Feachem, executive director of the Global Fund to Fight AIDS, Tuberculosis and Malaria (the Global

Fund), have all begged Canada to declare a timetable to reach 0.7 percent. Canada steadfastly refuses to do so.

Yet we are the only G8 country with successive and continuing budgetary surpluses. And our minister of finance, as a member of Blair's Commission on Africa, endorsed the target of 0.7 percent by 2015. It was the central recommendation of the commission report. How do you sign the report and then repudiate it upon your return to Canada? It's perverse; it lacks integrity.

We want to have it all ways. We declare our support for the crusade to "Make Poverty History"; we say we want to get to the 0.7 percent, but we resolutely refuse to set a timetable. The prime minister says that there's nothing worse in internationalism than to make promises that are not kept: that's the real immorality, he argues. With respect, he's wrong. The real immorality is for one of the most wealthy and privileged countries in the world to fail to respond adequately to the life and death struggle of hundreds of millions of impoverished people.

The irony is that on an issue like HIV/AIDS in the developing world, Canada's record is excellent. The reality is that our initiatives on the pandemic are completely eclipsed by our failure on foreign aid.

History will not judge our government kindly. In fact, we are not being judged kindly in the here and now. Just prior to the G8 Summit, the Human Development Report office of the UNDP issued its own survey on the performance of the G8 partners. It said in the first paragraph: "In the absence of a bold financing strategy, the Millennium Development Goals will be missed by a huge margin, especially in sub-Saharan Africa." It then did a country-by-country analysis, which was discouraging overall, with one key exception: "Of all the G8 countries, Canada is best placed to adopt and implement an ambitious target." But we're not headed in that direction. I repeat: History will not judge our government kindly.

I've put great emphasis on trade and debt and aid in this opening lecture for two reasons. First, these components effectively constitute the final and decisive MDG: "Develop a global partnership for development." Second, every other goal, without exception, is completely or significantly dependent on this one. There's no way around it. Unless we can summon a continuous flow of resources, the goals are doomed.

The particular focus on Official Development Assistance is also deliberate. While it is true that economic growth is ultimately tied to trade, there can be no sustained growth until the burden of disease is dealt with. It's a fatuous fantasy to think that whole populations, barely able physically to survive, can drive the economic engine. Restore health, and we'll restore hope for a robust economy. The two are inseparable. But it will never happen without a gigantic boost in foreign aid; it's foreign aid that gets ploughed into the social sectors, not private money, not foreign investment, not the dollars from commercial banks. If the promises of the G8 Summit fall apart, Africa falls apart with them. I may be a voice in isolation, but I'd be prepared to bet that the so-called doubling of aid by 2010 is as illusory as a mirage in the desert.

Early on in my tenure as envoy, I visited a little community centre, rundown, falling apart, but vibrant, in Kigali, Rwanda, where one or two hundred school children and their "caregivers" gathered at the end of each day for milk and cookies and play. The children were sitting on the lower steps of the compound's porch, and I was drawn to a trio of young girls. They turned out to be sisters, each of them consumed by shyness in the presence of a white visitor.

I bent down to talk with them, turning to the youngest, whom I found irresistible. She had the sweet, trusting face of a six-year-old, uncomfortably thin, very plain of feature, hair unkempt and straggled, but the entire portrait transformed by radiantly piercing green eyes. I asked about the parents: the father was dead, the mother was sick. I asked who looked after the girls: they looked after themselves. I asked if they went to school: they did occasionally when they didn't have to care for their mother.

The conversation was confined to that one little girl who answered me in whispers so muted that I had to place my ear almost to her lips to hear.

We finished talking, and I got up and walked the hundred yards or so to the far end of the compound, where the women caregivers had gathered in a raucous singing and dancing crowd to tell me about their grievances. They were tremendously animated and articulate, many of them HIV-positive, filled with predictable dread about what would happen to their children when they died.

I was standing just in front of them, asking questions, answering questions, when I suddenly felt a tiny figure tuck itself into my body, so close, so tight, it was as if we were welded one to the other. The little girl had come the full length of the compound just to seek the warmth of a friendly adult whom she did not know. I put my arms around her as we stood, locked together, and she followed the conversation with intensity, looking up at me every now and again with those eyes, those piercing green eyes.

The exchange with the mothers ended. I had to leave. I bent down and gently kissed the little girl on the cheek, and she looked at me, those eyes again looked at me, and they said it all: no accusation, just resignation. Another adult leaving her behind. It has become the story of the children of Africa.

I've never forgotten, and will never forget that encounter. I found the three sisters again a couple of years later. Miraculously, the mother was still alive, albeit ill. I shall try to see them again soon.

I wanted to do these lectures for all those little girls and all those mothers whose lives have been torn from their moorings, and whose future is in the hands, at least in part, of those who have always pretended to care, and have never really cared.

II

PANDEMIC: MY COUNTRY IS ON ITS KNEES

It will doubtless become clear, during the course of these lectures, that I have a love affair with Africa. It seems appropriate, therefore, to describe how that affair came about, and how it relates to the Africa of today.

I left the University of Toronto prematurely in the spring of 1960. It was premature because my academic career (a significant abuse of the word "career") was abysmal in the extreme, and when it became clear (it was never really in doubt) that I wouldn't graduate, I flunked out belligerently, and took off for other climes. I don't intend to search the depths of my psyche for an explanation, thus enlisting the bemusement of the Canadian public that may be listening to, or reading, these lectures. Suffice to say that I loved the university environment, feasted at its academic high tables, and read voraciously throughout my undergraduate years. But I just couldn't muster the energy for exams. It turned out to make little difference in life, although, if I may set your collective minds at ease, I don't wander around recommending similar conduct to the post-secondary youth of today.

My first job after university, in the early summer of 1960, was with the Socialist International in London, England. It seemed a perfect fit: it took me away from my hapless university career and allowed me, nonetheless, to follow my ideology. For those of you who may not be familiar with my ancestral political background, I was raised in a social democratic family: my father, David Lewis, was the federal secretary of the Co-operative Commonwealth Federation (CCF), precursor of the New Democratic Party (NDP), of which he eventually became the federal leader. I have a brother and two sisters; we all understood, even when pre-pubescent, that either we were ideological clones of our parents, or we were disinherited.

The Socialist International was a coordinating body of all of the democratic socialist parties in the western and developing world. It was defiantly anti-communist, and most member parties at the time would have described themselves as democrats first and socialists second. I was but a lowly researcher. However, simply being at the Socialist International allowed me a close-up view of both the British Labour Party and the British Trade Union movement. I was in England during the great Clause 4 debates on nationalization, which served me well in future years when I headed a provincial NDP caucus, some of whose members were maniacal public ownership fanatics.

My research role also permitted me to monitor mail on a daily basis. Lo and behold, after only a few weeks on the job, there fell into my hands an invitation, extended to all and sundry, to attend a week-long conference in September, of the World Assembly of Youth in Accra, Ghana. I was utterly intrigued and replied to say that I would be pleased to come to represent the hundreds of thousands of Canadian left-wing youth. (There were eight of us at the time.)

So off I went to Ghana, as thrilled and excited as any twenty-two-year-old would be at the prospect of adventure, however brief, on a new and, for me, unknown continent. Although the conference lasted only seven days, I stayed in Africa for a year; I was crazy about the continent from the moment I set foot on its soil — the music, the energy, the kindness, the generosity, the camaraderie, the purposefulness of everything. Remember, when I was in Ghana it had been independent for only two years; the sense of possibility was everywhere.

I found it all irresistible. The World Assembly of Youth was the best thing that had ever happened to me — so it was rather comical to learn several years later, via the poet-essayist-editor Stephen Spender in the pages of his monthly magazine, *Encounter*, that the World Assembly of Youth was a CIA front. I'm probably the first person you've ever met who's indebted to the CIA.

Ghana was a revelation in a number of ways. I had two jobs: teaching English and history at Accra High School, and "extra-mural studies" at the University of Legon. Just imagine, if you will, having *Merchant of Venice* as the Shakespeare text for a grade ten class, and fifteen minutes into a reading of the play, a bright young girl's hand goes up, and she asks with beatific innocence, "Mr. Lewis, what is a Jew?" I was momentarily stunned by the question. That innocence, that absence of malice, or prejudice, or intolerance (i.e., anti-Semitism) was one of the most heartwarming characteristics of the new Ghana — indeed, of all African countries in the immediate flowering of liberation.

My job at the University of Legon was even better than my daytime teaching job. I travelled three nights a week to villages within a fifty-kilometre radius of Accra, ferrying kerosene lamps and a portable library, teaching the literate elements of the community: the cocoa marketing board employees, the local teachers, the firefighters. It was giddy and exhilarating. They were desperate for learning, faces shining in the oscillating glimmer of the light. I can't remember when I've had such fun or been so excited by students.

But there was more. President Kwame Nkrumah — a pan-Africanist to his core; a man who saw a "United States of Africa" as the ultimate anti-colonial vindication of Africa's destiny — was flying South African dissidents in the dead of night out of what was then Basutoland (now Lesotho), a British protectorate surrounded by South Africa, and into the freedom of Ghana. This was the generation of freedom fighters yet to come, and they stayed in student residences on the Legon campus. I became fast friends with many of them and soaked up the anti-apartheid liberation ideology. It was particularly easy to do because also living on the campus, having recently been thrown out of South Africa by then president Hendrik Verwoerd, was Leslie Rubin. When Alan Paton (the celebrated author of *Cry, the Beloved Country*) was president, Leslie had been vice-president of the Liberal Party, serving as the last elected white person representing Africans of the Cape Province in the South African senate. Those were the grounds for his eviction by Verwoerd.

I worshipped Leslie; we spent a great deal of time together during the few months I was in Ghana. After he left South Africa, he became the first dean of the University of Legon Law School, later authoring the definitive Ghanaian constitution. He was a kind and fatherly figure, a man of great principle and passion in the anti-apartheid struggle. Apart from his natural academic gifts, Leslie was a pamphleteer of extraordinary talent, often writing under the pseudonym of Martin Burger, savaging the apartheid administration. His finest tract, which had great influence outside of South Africa, was titled "This Is Apartheid," and consisted of a remarkably down-to-earth, non-legal, populist exposition of forty apartheid laws. It was a truly blood-chilling document, exposing for all the world to see the madness and brutality of the Nazi-like regime.

One of the bizarre consequences of these varied and valued contacts in Ghana was a phone call my father received in the fall of 1960, out of the blue, from the Canadian Ministry of Foreign Affairs, saying that I had been banned from South Africa. My father couldn't figure out how that had happened when his son was clearly resident in Ghana, but he soon understood: one of the well-known incidental truths about apartheid was its twisted and demented irrationality. I was *persona non grata* by association, and it was particularly absurd because of course I had not the slightest intention of visiting South Africa. However, the encounters with my new South African friends, and their tales of ugly fascism at home had an influence on me which lasted for the rest of my life. It was no accident that when I was elected to the Ontario Legislature in 1963, one of my earliest private member's bills was an act designed to ban the import of South African wines and liquors into Ontario. Many of my legislative colleagues were mystified; my Tory friends were derisive. But my views had been well and truly formed.

I had been in Ghana for just a few months when I received a letter from a young man I'd met at the World Assembly of Youth, Mokwugo Okoye, a radical left-wing activist living in what was the Eastern Region in Nigeria. He wrote to say that a Peace Corps volunteer slated to be the principal of a little private boarding secondary school in Mok's village had failed to turn up, and was I interested in coming to Nigeria to fill the post? How could I say no? In early 1961, I drove several hundred kilometres to the Eastern Region, taking up residence in a tiny village between the regional capital, Enugu, and the hub of commercial activity, the chaotic city of Onitsha.

Mok was an astonishing figure. He was a polemicist of raging voice and pen, much admired throughout the country for his intense nationalism and formidable literary power. He was just a few years older than I, and patiently schooled me in the perplexing, often incomprehensible minutiae of Nigerian politics, all of which would serve me well in later life. My sojourn at the school was equally compelling. It had but four classes — two grade nines, two grade tens — with a total student body of about one hundred. I loved those kids: they were so anxious to learn, so excited by the potential reach of knowledge that every class was thrilling, for them and for me. A boarding school allows for a special camaraderie, with teachers and students on a shared site: the sense of family was very real. One of the saddest, most wretched experiences of my life, was to return to the Eastern Region, during the Biafran civil war in the late 1960s, to try to find my former students, only to discover that many of them had died — some from bullets, some from hunger, some from both. It proved to be a premonitory glimpse of things to come.

After several exhilarating months in Nigeria, I asked a Canadian friend to join me, and we drove together across the continent through Chad, the Central African Republic, the Congo, Sudan, Uganda and, finally, Kenya. (It took us about five weeks; it was not supposed to be possible.) I taught trade unionists in Uganda at the International Confederation of Free Trade Unions' African Labour College in Kampala, and ended up in Nairobi in a job that involved finding university places in North America for African students.

It was in August 1961 that I received a letter from Tommy Douglas, asking me to return to Canada to work for the very recently formed New Democratic Party. I accepted his invitation to leap back into Canada's political fray with abiding reluctance. (You couldn't say no to Tommy, the same Tommy Douglas who that very month in 1961 had become the first leader of the NDP, and was recently chosen in the CBC poll as the greatest Canadian of them all.) On my return to Canada in the fall, I plunged into excited pre-election activity as the first full-time federal organizer for the NDP.

It was, however, incredibly hard to say goodbye to Africa. I travelled there again in the late 1960s, and returned, with regularity, when I was a Canadian diplomat at the United Nations, then with UNICEF, and finally, now, as the HIV/AIDS envoy. I have spent time, at one point or another, in the great majority of the countries on the continent.

It must be understood, without any hint of heady romanticism, that Africa in the 1950s and 1960s, when I was most impressionable, was a continent of vitality, growth, and boundless expectation. It got into your blood, your viscera, your heart. The bonds were not just durable, they were unbreakable. There was something intoxicating about an environment of such hope, anticipation, affection, energy, indomitability. The Africa I knew was poor, but it wasn't staggering under the weight of oppression, disease, and despair; it was absolutely certain that it could triumph over every exigency. There were countless health emergencies — polio, measles, malaria, malnutrition — but it never felt like Armageddon. In fact, life expectancy began to rise in the late 1960s, until the reversal induced by Structural Adjustment Programs on the one hand, and AIDS on the other. And the people, the people everywhere, were so unbelievably kind; I had never encountered cultures so uniformly inclusive, gentle, decent, welcoming.

I was smitten for life.

You can understand, therefore, how painful it is to visit my beloved Africa under present-day circumstances. It's not just the ruinous economic and social decline, the reasons for which I attempted to explain in part in my first lecture. It's the ravaging of the pandemic; it's the way in which a communicable disease called AIDS has taken countries by the throat and reduced them to spectral caricatures of their former selves.

It's impossible to write about the Millennium Development Goals without writing about HIV/AIDS, and that's not simply because defeating the pandemic is one of those goals. It's because every goal, at least in Africa, is put in jeopardy by AIDS. I remember sitting in the General Assembly on June 2, 2005, when there was a Special Session to assess the progress that had been made since the Declaration of Commitment on AIDS was embraced, by consensus, at a more elaborate UN gathering in 2001. Rather mournfully, the Secretary-General told the assembled delegates that progress was minimal, that most countries had defaulted on their commitments, that the pandemic was outpacing the response, and that the MDGS were thus imperiled.

Later that day, at a press conference, Peter Piot, the executive director of UNAIDS, was far less guarded. He said, flatly, that the goals would not be reached.

There is just no way to compare the Africa of forty-five years ago with the Africa of today. It's like comparing Rome with Pompeii. So let me tell you, by way of a procession of anecdotes, what Pompeii looks like. I've deliberately chosen anecdotes as the narrative vehicle, in order to give the pandemic an accessible face, rather than relying on the dehumanizing swamp of numbers. Some of the stories you may have heard before, but all illumine an aspect of Africa's desperation. I don't pretend that every country is similarly afflicted. Southern Africa is the terrifying epicentre, East Africa, including Ethiopia, is in serious straits, central Africa is struggling, and only West Africa seems able to contain the virus. But even there, in countries like Nigeria, Côte d'Ivoire, Cameroon, and Burkina Faso, huge numbers of people are infected or at risk.

It was 2002; I was visiting the Lilongwe Central Hospital in the capital of Malawi. The adult medical wards, male and female, presented a picture right out of Dante. There were two people to every bed, head to foot and foot to head, and in most instances, someone under the bed on the concrete floor, each in an agony of full-blown AIDS. With demonic, rhythmic regularity, another aluminum coffin would be wheeled into the ward to cart away the body of the person who had most recently died.

Every patient was a near cadaver. The wards rumbled with low, almost-inaudible moans, as though those who were ill could not summon the strength to give voice to the pain. The smell was awful: a room of rotting feces and stale urine. And the eyes, so sunken and glazed and pleading.

I talked with the administrator. He told me that on the ten-hour night shift, to care for between sixty and seventy patients — each and every one of whom would have been in intensive care in a Canadian hospital — there would be one nurse. The situation was impossible.

But the situation is impossible in much of southern Africa. The pandemic has taken a decimating toll on nurses, doctors, and clinicians of every variety. There are simply no pharmacists to speak of; incredible though it may seem, I can't remember a hospital or clinic that had a full-time pharmacist. You might well ask: Who, then, dispenses the antiretroviral drugs for the treatment of AIDS? The answer is: Anyone who can be found. The pandemic has also ravaged the ranks of community health workers, teachers, farmers — absolutely every professional discipline, every occupation.

The problem is grievously compounded by the practice of "poaching," and the resulting brain drain from Africa to the outside world. Some of the drain goes to other countries in the region — South Africa or Botswana, for example — but they, too, lose professionals in the predominant flow to the United Kingdom, the United States, Australia, and Canada. It's rancid behaviour on the part of the West.

Please don't misunderstand me. People have the human right to move to better jobs, with better pay, better benefits, better working conditions. But given the situation in Africa, they shouldn't be induced to leave by countries perfectly capable of solving occupational deficits internally. The United Kingdom in particular has a dreadful record; it's said — and not in jest — that there are more Malawian doctors in Manchester than in Malawi, more Zambian doctors in Birmingham than in Zambia. When confronted with these facts, the U.K. government replies by saying that they've passed a law which forbids any public health facility in the United Kingdom from the solicitation of health-care workers in developing countries. And that is indeed the case. What they don't acknowledge, however, is the real problem: personnel agencies advertise for professional people, travelling to the countries of southern Africa and interviewing potential candidates, and offering all manner of monetary and related incentives. Until the personnel agencies are barred from such shameless raiding, the protestations of western governments — all of which, to a lesser or greater degree, turn a blind eye — ring hollow.

The other remedy, of course, is to provide significant salary increases for professionals who remain at home, improvements in working conditions, expanded training of health professionals, and even the creation of new career lines — adequate to do the job, but requiring less by way of formal accreditation. The U.K.'s international development agency has a pilot project with exactly those components underway in Malawi; would that it became the pattern across the continent.

The loss of health-care personnel has become a crisis of huge proportions. But it is only one of many crises which turn so many countries on the continent into a quagmire of despair.

In 2003, I had the privilege of travelling in Zambia and Uganda with Graça Machel, a good friend (and hero) of mine with whom I have worked, intermittently, over the last decade. Graça is the former minister of education of Mozambique, the former first lady of Mozambique, now married to Nelson Mandela, and known everywhere in Africa as one of the most charismatic and compelling of personalities. She is also gentle, generous, formidably intelligent, and profoundly knowledgeable about the African continent. Together we wanted to examine the situation of women and children in the face of the pandemic.

In Uganda we experienced two telling episodes. We were taken to ground zero of the pandemic, the district of Rakai, where the first case of HIV was diagnosed in 1982. The local community very much wanted us to see what was happening to the orphans, and in the first instance we were led to a large hut and escorted inside. Immediately to the left of the door as we entered, sat the patriarch of the family, eighty-six years old, clutching a white cane, entirely blind. To the right of the door sat his two wives, one seventy-six, the other seventy-eight. Between them they had given birth to nine children, eight of whom were dead. The ninth was visibly dying in our presence. In the interior of the hut, the orphans had gathered, and sitting on the floor, looking up at us expectantly, were thirty-six orphan children between the ages of two and sixteen.

Graça and I exchanged those wordless glances that occur between adults when there's a feeling of helplessness in the air. Just how the two grandmothers were supposed to cope under the circumstances was nowhere evident. The older kids were out of school because they couldn't afford the school fees, and the younger kids were surviving on one meal a day, or sometimes no food whatsoever on the weekends.

It leads me to want to say a word about grandmothers. They have emerged as the heroes of Africa. The physical ravaging of extended families and the desperate poverty of communities means that grandmothers step in when there's no one else to tread. I wonder if such a situation has ever occurred before in the history of organized society? I wish there were more authoritative information about what happened to orphans during the Black Death of the fourteenth century.

In the instance of Africa today, these old and unimaginably frail women often look after five or ten or fifteen kids, enduring every conceivable hardship for the sake of their grandchildren, alongside additional numbers of other abandoned waifs who wander the landscape of the continent. The trauma of the grandmothers equals that of the orphans; in fact, every normal rhythm of life is violated as grandmothers bury their own children and then look after their orphan grandchildren. I remember, vividly, sitting under the trees, outside the Alex/Tara Children's Clinic in Alexandra Township in Johannesburg, with about twenty grandmothers as they told their heartbreaking stories of personal loss, one by one. I could barely imagine how they were functioning; every one of them had made that heart-wrenching trek to the graveyard, many more than once, and yet they spoke with a spunk and resilience that was positively supernatural.

Save one. There was one woman, seventy-three years old, sitting slightly apart from the rest, who refused to speak. No amount of encouragement or cajoling would do, until the women collectively, in an incredibly moving show of commiseration, sang a soft song of solidarity and love.

And then Agnes finally spoke. She took no more than a couple of minutes: her story was wrenchingly brief, ghastly in its simplicity. She had buried all five of her adult children between 2001 and 2003 — all five — and was left with four orphan grandchildren. That was it. She wept.

I learned as I left that every one of her four grandchildren is HIV-positive. How much can one grandmother endure?

But alas, that's not the end of it. When the grandmothers die, there's no one coming up behind, and so you have the phenomenon of what we call "child-headed households," or "sibling families," where the oldest child is the head of the household, looking after his or her siblings. It's not new: it happened in Rwanda after the genocide. But never have we had a situation involving such large numbers. In Zambia, 23 percent of all children are orphans now, with numbers expected to rise to one in three by 2010; inevitably, a significant number will find themselves in sibling families. In Swaziland, it's expected that up to 15 percent of the entire population will be orphans by 2010. I well remember meeting with several members of the Swaziland cabinet, discussing matters of public policy, when the minister of labour suddenly jumped to his feet, impatient and agitated. "Forget about this policy stuff," he said, his voice rising. "Don't you understand that we're a nation of orphans? That we have hundreds of child-headed households in Swaziland, where the age of the child heading the household is eight?"

Back in Uganda, Graça and I were taken by the local villagers to see one of those sibling families. There were five children in all: three girls, 14, 12 and 10, and two boys, 11 and 8. We entered the modest hut, and sat down with our backs to the wall, Graça with her arm around the three girls on her right and I with my arm around the two boys on my left. Graça then told all the hangers-on to leave — all the media, all the UN staff — except for one community worker and one translator.

I had no idea what was coming. Graça turned to the two older girls, and in a most gentle, reassuring voice asked, "Have you started to menstruate yet?" The two girls, clearly startled, replied in those shy, barely audible whispered voices so characteristic of African children, "Yes." Then Graça began to ask a series of questions: "Do you know what it means? Have you talked to anyone about it? Do you talk to the villagers about it — your teachers, your fellow students? Does anyone bring you any pads?"

The atmosphere was intense, the little girls, now fully embraced in Graça's arms, seemed to have suspended breathing, and I suddenly understood that I was witness to the first act of "mothering" that these girls had ever received about one of the most transfiguring experiences of a young girl's life.

I've told this story a number of times because the experience had a profound impact on me. At the moment when Graça asked her questions, I thought to myself: That's what's happening right across the continent: the transfer of love and knowledge and values and experience from one generation to the next is gone, and with it goes the confidence and security and sense of place which children normally take for granted. Children, already traumatized by the death of their parents, are left reeling as they confront the void in the aftermath.

As we were leaving, I asked the oldest sister, "Who puts you to bed at night?"

"I put everyone to bed," she replied.

"But bedtime can be pretty scary," I offered. "The nights are dark, the dreams can be upsetting. Don't any of the neighbours come in to help?"

"No," she said, matter-of-factly. "I put them to bed myself. I'm the mother."

I can't emphasize strongly enough the extreme emotional turmoil of children orphaned by AIDS. What the world fails to recognize is that these children don't become orphans when their parents die, they become orphans while their parents are dying, and this is especially true in the case of the death of the mother.

I've now seen innumerable people die, in hospital wards, in clinic corridors, in hospices, and at home. When they die at home, the scene — almost Shakespearean in its sense of tragedy and finality interwoven — is invariably the same. I'm taken to a tiny rural village to see the application of "home-based care." I enter a hut, where the bleakness and gloom are palpable. On the floor of the hut lies a young woman — always young — in her twenties or thirties, so wan and emaciated as to be unable to lift either hand or head. I bend down, painfully inadequate to the circumstance, and touch her brow, uttering some pointless banality which is intended to soothe, and then as I step back, looking around me, I see her children, all her children, standing in the darkened shadows, watching their mother die.

How do they ever recover? The death is long, agonizing, and filled with indignity. The children wash their mother, they clean her up when she's incontinent (an experience of excruciating embarrassment for both mother and children), they search everywhere for an aspirin to relieve the pain of some opportunistic infection, and then, horrified, gaping, they stand in the darkened shadows, and watch their mother die.

There is, undoubtedly, some solace to be found in the comfort of relatives, if relatives exist, especially grandmothers, if they're still alive. But as I write, there is no master plan for children orphaned by AIDS. There are to be sure, as there always are, endless studies, and individual projects and frameworks. But nothing is yet taken to scale. The gap between analysis and action yawns like the proverbial chasm, and it's only now, in 2005, a quarter century into the pandemic, that we're beginning to think of a response to the orphans. I shall try to deal with what should be done in my final lecture.

There are certain other aspects of the pandemic that I should like to reconnoitre to demonstrate the contrast between the conditions of today and the conditions of yesteryear.

The first is surprising: it's the monumental crisis of food. I can't remember, when I travelled through the continent forty-five years ago, encountering families, let alone whole communities, who were hungry. I'm sure they existed: I just didn't encounter them. By and large, there was always enough food for everyone; poverty was ubiquitous, but it didn't mean starvation.

Whenever I travel in Africa today, it feels as though everyone is hungry — hungry to the point of starvation. There are, certainly, very real areas of famine — Zimbabwe, Zambia, Malawi, Lesotho, Swaziland, Mozambique — they have all suffered terrible droughts over the last several years, and the drought cum pandemic have added up to starvation. But it's more than that. It's hard to go anywhere on the continent without people crying out for food. In fact, if you ask almost anyone what they need most, including people suffering from full-blown AIDS, they will not say drugs; they will say food. It's a universal reply.

I recall visiting with a large group of widows and grandmothers in a rural community hall in Malawi (coincidentally called Canada Hall, with a blurred Canadian flag on the wall because it had been built with Canadian aid money) to chat with them about their lives in the midst of the virus. The conversation was dominated — totally dominated — by pleas for food. It was incomparably sad; I had no food to give them, but that's all they really wanted of me. Sure, I steered things into talk of treatment, and at one point, even tried to raise the issue of condoms, but every voice came back to food. It's so stark and so troubling: even though there was an interpreter present so that no words were lost, the women constantly pointed at their mouths and stomachs to make absolutely sure that I wouldn't miss what agitated them most.

The question of hunger becomes so much more critical in the presence of AIDS. Treatment is much more difficult, sometimes impossible, if the patient has nothing to eat: the body can't handle the drugs without food. And the further bitter truth is that full-blown AIDS can sometimes be forestalled for a considerable period of time if the body is receiving nutritious foods. When I was in Malawi, I kept repeating the defining mantra: If the body has no food to consume, the virus consumes the body.

I'm not sure there is an answer to this debilitating and systemic plague of hunger, but I shall try to suggest a response as I wind my way to the end of the lectures.

Certainly when I travelled forty-five years ago, death was never a constant companion. But in the presence of the pandemic, it sometimes feels as though death stalks every waking moment. And as the four years of my work have unfolded, more and more it's the death of older children and young adults that is so widespread, stark and unnerving.

I shall inevitably talk a lot about death in these lectures, but let me be intensely personal about it for a moment. I was completely unprepared for the pervasiveness of death. It has shaken me to my core. I must admit that from time to time the enveloping cloak of death, combined with the appalling paucity of response has made me feel futile in the face of the pandemic. I never submit to those momentary lapses because futility leads nowhere, but the way in which death seeps into every crevice of life shifts one's view of the world. I'm not sure I can even find the words to explain it: all of us who live in privileged western societies experience death from time to time, but in much of southern Africa that's all people know. Their lives consist of attending funerals; if I may mangle a phrase, they go on a graveyard crawl every weekend. It's commonplace to say that every family in every country — Kenya, Uganda, Tanzania, Zimbabwe, Zambia, Malawi, Lesotho, Swaziland, South Africa, Namibia, Mozambique, Botswana — has suffered a loss in the carnage of AIDS. But merely to use the words is to rob them of meaning.

One of the moments that lives most ineradicably in my mind, occurred during a visit to the pediatric ward of the University Teaching Hospital in Lusaka, Zambia, in 2003. It was at the height of famine, and every crib had four or five infants and toddlers crushed together between the raised slatted sides, most of them suffering extreme malnutrition or AIDS or both. Their bodies were so thin that it was legitimate to ask, how can they still be alive?

Well, as it happens, not all of them were. Approximately ten minutes into the visit, the walls of the ward vibrated with what can only be called an other-worldly wail — a wail the like of which I had never before heard. I was stunned, and convulsively spun around to find the source. There, kneeling by the side of a bed, embodying anguish and despair, rocking violently back and forth, was a young mother crazed by loss, watching a nurse firmly place a sheet over the body of an infant and take the child away.

Incredible though it may seem, the exact episode was twice more repeated during my forty minutes in the ward. It prompted no brake on the pace of activity; it was commonplace. In the pediatric ward of the University Teaching Hospital in Lusaka, Zambia, throughout 2003, nothing was more commonplace than death.

I remember visiting the wonderful little faith-based organization called Catholic AIDS Action in Windhoek, Namibia. It is a place where people living with AIDS come together to network and seek companionable solace. Sister Raphaele excitedly showed me around, and then asked if I'd go out back to see their income-generating project. I did so, and was greeted by the sight of four young men making miniature papier mâché coffins for infants: tiny, light, plain. As they affixed silver aluminum foil handles to the coffins, they looked at me and said, with an admixture of pride and pain, "We can't keep up with the demand."

I'm reminded of another "income-generating" project, this time in Zambia. It was early in 2005, and I was asked by a district commissioner to visit a fairly remote farming community where a group of village women had a project of which they were greatly proud.

We rode in our Land Rovers over some hideously rocky and tortuous country roads, and then had to get out and walk a fair bit further. Eventually we came to a large cabbage patch, beside which stood a group of fifteen or twenty women holding aloft a large banner reading "PLWA," proclaiming their status as People Living With AIDS.

After several minutes of animated conversation, I asked if the cabbages were the project (not a brilliant hunch on my part). They laughed uproariously and said yes. "You use it to supplement your diet?" Yes again. "Do you have a surplus?"

"Yes," they chorused, "We take whatever we don't use to market."

"And what do you do with the profit?" I asked. It was here that time stood still. They looked at me for ages, as though I were asking a question to which I surely knew the answer, and then they suddenly realized that the question was genuine. "We buy coffins of course," they said. "We never have enough coffins."

My mind ricocheted back to Catholic AIDS Action: "We can't keep up with the demand."

There is just no way to convey the atmosphere of death which hangs like a Damoclean *hammer* over these countries. I have heard the president of Botswana use the word "extermination" to describe what he feels his country is dealing with. I have heard the prime minister of Lesotho use the word "annihilation" to describe what he feels his country is confronting. In my last close conversation with the president of Zambia, he used the word "holocaust" to describe what he feels his country is facing. In June 2005, the new deputy prime minister of

Namibia said publicly that her country was "on its knees."

It's heartbreaking to see the Africa I once knew reduced to such desperation.

And death comes with such terrifying speed. When I first travelled to Zambia in the envoy role in 2001, I met the most wonderful group of PLWAS. There must have been twenty, most of them young women — bright, engaging young women; we sat around a large table in a hotel conference room as they laid out their concerns and grievances. They were so smart and so lively, and I loved the conversation. Eight months later I went back to Zambia and met with the group again, and more than half of them were gone. I was afraid to enquire about the absentees because I knew, all too well, why they were absent.

It's actually a pattern. A couple of years back, I met with eighteen representatives of various district and regional groups of PLWAS in Rwanda. They told me that they had met the year previous with UNAIDS Executive Director Peter Piot. Sixteen of the eighteen who had met with Peter were not alive to meet with me.

It's so incredibly painful. You make friends and the friends are gone before you can consummate the friendship. These groups of people living with AIDS are remarkably courageous, coming forward, declaring their status, preaching the message of prevention, sustaining each other in the face of cosmic tragedy. And yet they're scorned and mocked by government, and rarely listened to, rarely given an audience with the powers-that-be. Worse, society heaps endless, often brutal, sometimes even murderous stigma and discrimination upon those who are infected. The antagonism comes from intimate family, from friends, from fellow workers, from teachers, from clerics — no one escapes the barbs and malice. Even the children are targets, mocked and stoned on the way home from school.

It would be wrong, however, and in a sense too easy, to conjure up only the pictures of despair. Let me recount some of the images of hope, because it's the images of hope, however fragile, however intermittent, that keep the countries going.

I was visiting the southern province of Ethiopia in 2004. In the little town of Nazareth, the UN's World Food Programme (WFP), had gathered together a large contingent of truck drivers, two hundred strong, who had undergone a training course on HIV prevention. The idea was smart and it was logical. These were the drivers who encountered commercial sex workers along their delivery routes, the truck drivers whom we regularly list in the high-risk-group category, the truck drivers who return to their homes and partners and spread the virus. So the WFP had conducted workshops on prevention, and I turned out to be the visitor with whom their stories could be shared.

It was memorable and it was hilarious, rather like a robust church service of confessions. One by one these hardy men straggled to the front of the room to give personal testimony. Strangled by unaccustomed shyness, each and every one, they described how they use condoms at every sexual encounter, and would never again venture forth without a supply of condoms (judiciously supplied, free of charge, by the WFP). There was much merriment, much embarrassment, much applause.

And then one of the only two women in the room muscled her way to the front, ostentatiously pushing the men aside. To roars of approval, she announced that it was all true: she knew that the men really did carry condoms, and used them whenever the need arose. She was an itinerant trucker, but also a local organizer, and clearly knew whereof she spoke. It was one of those moments to be cherished. The World Food Programme staff were justly proud of their success.

That reminds me of an encounter involving the other side of the equation. The city of Nairobi, on its outskirts, is home to Kibera, possibly the worst slum in all of East Africa. There are large numbers of commercial sex workers, most of whom are part of a little community-based organization run by Professor Elizabeth Ngugi, who teaches community medicine at the University of Nairobi.

Elizabeth Ngugi is a force of nature. She's a diminutive sixty-seven-year-old, of irrepressible energy and a speaking style reminiscent of the grand orators of yore. She took me to the headquarters of the commercial sex workers' group, where about a hundred had gathered. There she launched into a cascading torrent of speechifying, the like of which I haven't heard anywhere else in Africa. Despite the demagogic quality — or perhaps because of it — the women began to sing in their local language, and to dance, wildly waving unopened condoms above their heads. The song apparently conveyed their unanimous commitment to using condoms for the rest of their lives.

It was a wonderfully raucous scene. And then I asked Elizabeth, *sotto voce*, what percentage of the women she thought were HIV-positive. "About 80 percent," was her unhesitating reply. By now I suspect that most of them will have "passed" (the East African term for "died"), but at least the men with whom they had protected sex will not be infected.

It was so supremely sad and so exhilarating in equal measure.

Let me transport you to Lusaka, Zambia, and a remarkable residential school for girls called Umoyo. The school has sixty students, all between the ages of fifteen and nineteen, all chosen by their respective communities (called "compounds" in Lusaka), and all of them orphaned by AIDS. The school itself has a good teacher–student ratio, and the staff members are uniformly first-rate. The principal is a male feminist of strong conviction. The entire atmosphere is resolute and loving.

The girls spend the first month or two recovering from the trauma of parental death; it's a pretty scary, emotionally volatile time. The next couple of months consist of acclimatizing to each other, with all of the rambunctious swings of mood and behaviour that characterize the teenage years. The final eight months or so are an immersion in academe, and these young women invariably score as high on country-wide tests as any group of young people in any regular school.

I have to say that I have yet to visit any other learning environment in southern Africa that does a better job of girls' empowerment. Somehow, the devotion and affection suffusing the school transmits itself to the girls, and they emerge as an immensely appealing, irrepressible, and bright group of young women. They like each other immensely, and they draw both strength and camaraderie from the intense, shared experience.

I visited Umoyo on two particularly memorable occasions, once with Graça Machel, and once with none other than Oprah Winfrey. Graça was so bowled over by the girls that she vowed to come back for their graduation. Oprah was bowled over, period; she clearly cherished the encounter.

And these encounters are indeed something to behold. The girls burst into song and rhythmic dance at the sight of visitors, their voices meshed in soaring crescendo, so exquisitely musical, so energetic, so joyous that you'd never guess at the tragedy that lurks beneath. And then, when you start to ask questions, as we all did, the self-confidence and brazen candour take your breath away. These are young women who will never automatically submit to any young man; young women who will insist that a condom be worn; young women who will report sexual violence; young women who will stay and work in their own communities. Every one of them learns a trade at Umoyo, sometimes tailoring, sometimes food preparation, sometimes carpentry, sometimes hair-dressing — the nature of the trade matters not. They feel confident that when they leave Umoyo, they'll succeed, and overwhelmingly, they do.

The entire program is a testament to possibilities — possibilities that speak to hope in the face of so much desolation. Fifteen to nineteen is the age group most vulnerable to the virus: Umoyo proves that prevention consists of far more than life skills classes, or cleverly constructed learning modules; it consists of the kind of affirmative action for girls that undoes all the cumulative damage done over time, to their perceptions of themselves, their egos, their self-confidence, their sexuality.

So, too, treatment. There are two anecdotes from Uganda which speak volumes. Graça and I visited the Mulago Hospital in Kampala — specifically, its clinic for pregnant women enrolled in a program called "PMTCT," which stands for "Prevention of Mother-to-Child Transmission." (Do you see how everything, even language, conspires against the woman? How is it that we choose an acronym that avoids the question of who infected the mother?)

It's the unhappy truth that only 5 to 8 percent of pregnant women in sub-Saharan Africa have access to programs of PMTCT. This is a terrible deficiency; there is no excuse for this state of affairs. Because of the low access rates, thousands upon thousands of babies are born HIV-positive who need not be infected; most of them die — helplessly, pathetically — before the age of two. But for those HIV-positive women who have access to PMTCT, the program is a godsend: when infected mothers-to-be take one tablet of the wonder drug nevirapine during the birthing process, and their newborns are given a liquid equivalent within seventy-two hours of birth, the rate of transmission is cut by up to 53 percent.

Of course, if we were to use the practices employed in the western world — that is to say, full antiretroviral therapy for the HIV-positive mother for the final twenty-four weeks of pregnancy — we'd be talking of a transmission rate of 1 or 2 percent! Such is the curse of double standards. It's a true obscenity that all those little lives are lost because the resources aren't available to provide a standard of care routinely offered in industrial countries.

However, the better news is that soon after it was introduced in Africa, PMTCT morphed into PMTCT-*Plus*, where the *Plus* represents treatment of the mother, her partner, and the family.

And therein lies a tale. I vividly remember standing outside a little PMTCT clinic in Kigali, Rwanda, back in 2002, chatting with three pregnant women who had tested HIV-positive and decided to take nevirapine. They were in high good spirits, and put to me quite strongly the following proposition: "Mr. Lewis, we'll do anything to save our children, but what about us?" The question could not have been more apt. It's obviously wonderful to save the child, but why should we then lose the mother?

Enter an innovative consortium of American foundations, led by the Rockefeller Foundation. They collectively decided to initiate a program of PMTCT-*Plus* at a number of facilities across the continent, directed overall by the Columbia School of Public Health. It is now in place, and it is working. And the proof that it's working was exemplified, dramatically, at that little pregnancy clinic at the Mulago hospital.

Some words of medical jargon are now required. In Africa, when the CD4 count of an infected person falls below two hundred, that person requires treatment. The CD4 count is a measure of certain white blood cells. I have seen people with CD4 counts of one hundred, fifty, thirty, even twenty, and when they go on treatment, they experience the Lazarus effect: they're at death's door, and the antiretroviral drugs literally bring them back to life, often in a matter of weeks.

In the waiting-room of the Mulago clinic, Graça and I met a women whose CD4 count had dropped to *one*. I have no idea how she was still alive. But the doctors had determined they would try treatment, despite so grim a prognosis, and the results were miraculous. So there she was, three months later, smiling exultantly, her HIV-negative baby in her lap, and, playing at her feet, her two other young children.

You see, it can be done. If only the world were to care, Africa can be brought back to the life it once had.

Another evocative excursion within Uganda, this one in 2004, took me to the northwest corner of the country, to the little town of Arua, where Médecins Sans Frontières (MSF, also known as Doctors Without Borders) had set up shop at the local hospital two years earlier. It has to be said that MSF is one of the most impressive NGOS anywhere: principled, effective, radical. They not only do an excellent humanitarian job, saving lives wherever they intervene, but they also brook no nonsense from either national or external governments. On many issues, they are more outspoken than any other leading member of civil society.

On this occasion, I had travelled north in the company of Uganda's minister of health to celebrate the second anniversary of MSF's opening of a treatment program in Arua, where previously treatment had been a pipe dream. As always, MSF had done a remarkable job. There were eleven hundred people in treatment already, twenty-five hundred more on a list for future treatment, and an atmosphere of irrepressible joy cascading through the surrounding community.

Nothing could contain the sense of community exuberance. Across the sprawling grounds of the hospital, one group after another came forward to join in the noisy celebration: women living with AIDS, Muslim women living with AIDS (certainly a first for me), men living with AIDS (also a first for me, as a group separate from women), and a deliciously rowdy contingent of people living with AIDS from across the border in the Democratic Republic of the Congo. There was a boisterous parade through town, accompanied by marching bands, and then everyone — perhaps a couple of thousand — repaired to the hospital for the panorama of speeches, dancing, drama, drums, song, and poetry. It's doubtful that spirits could have soared any higher.

As I stood there drinking it all in, I suddenly realized a startling truth: there was no stigma! The universal availability of free treatment and HIV counseling in Arua meant that the population had nothing to hide. MSF had achieved a near-miracle: keeping people alive on the one hand, and routing stigma and discrimination on the other. It was tremendously inspiring to see so many infected people moving confidently, casually, proudly through the throngs, without the corrosive backlash of prejudice and intolerance.

It will be a long, long time before that experience becomes commonplace in Africa. MSF has only so many professionals, and while the MSF models are exemplary, there are only a relative handful of them across the continent. Stigma is the bane of progress; it savages and ravages, ostracizes and isolates those who are living with the virus. Eradicating stigma will be the last holdout in the epic battle against AIDS.

Still, the little community of Arua gives a glimpse of what might be. I believe to the depths of my being that Africa will one day rejoice in a time when families are whole and funerals are rare. It's just so bitter that such multitudes of lives are being lost along the way. It's hard not to be in a near stupor of anger. And yet I'm sustained, as so many Africans are, by the memories of what the continent used to be, and the conviction that the present will one day reunite with the best of the past.

III

EDUCATION: AN AVALANCHE OF STUDIES, LITTLE STUDYING

IN MARCH OF 2002, I made a trip to Ethiopia which had one particularly memorable encounter. On an early morning, in the new conference centre in Addis Ababa, I met with nearly a thousand students, late primary and high school age, for a question-and-answer session on HIV/AIDS that lasted more than two hours. I began with a few opening remarks, and then the questions poured forth. The students were completely unselfconscious: they heckled each other energetically, laughed uproariously, and addressed matters of intimate sexuality as if they were in private conversation with an imported therapist.

I would not have anticipated it, but what concerned them most was the reliability of condoms. Clearly influenced by what they'd heard from both the Ethiopian Orthodox and Catholic churches, they pressed me hard on whether condoms were 35 percent or 50 percent or 95 percent effective. When I assured them that condoms were one of the absolutely most reliable means to prevent infection, and if they were sexually active, they must use condoms (boisterous applause at this point, signifying approval for sexual activity, I think, rather than condom use), my words were accepted without challenge. They were clearly relieved. It became evident, during the course of the two hours, that what the students wanted was reliable information that they could trust. They spoke warmly of their teachers, but they wanted corroboration of what their teachers had told them. They were irrepressibly voluble; they asked question after question, minds and spirits fully engaged.

I found it exhilarating. The best moment came right at the end, in an unexpected way. A young girl — she couldn't have been more than fourteen — sitting squarely in the front row, speaking with a strong, clear voice that resonated through the hall, said to me, "Sir, I don't want to have sex. The boys want me to have sex, but I refuse. They laugh at me behind my back, and they make fun of me in school. They say I'm stupid. I have a question: Do you think it's stupid to want to stay alive?"

Somewhere the proverbial pin dropped. And then there was slow, rhythmic clapping, ending in thunderous applause. And the thousand kids gave that young girl a standing ovation. I didn't have to say a word. But I remember thinking to myself how wonderful it was, in the midst of the chaos of the pandemic, to have access to education, to have young minds with the opportunity to grapple with so many difficult issues, with matters of life and death.

All of which prompts me to frame these remarks with education at the centre, and Ethiopia, coincidentally, as the takeoff point. You may remember that in my first lecture, I mentioned the African Development Forum. It was launched in the year 2000, under the auspices of the Economic Commission for Africa, based in Addis Ababa, where all subsequent forums would be held. The intent of the African Development Forum was to bring a wide cross-section of African leaders and activists together, on an annual basis, to discuss subjects of intense interest to the continent. The inaugural conference in 2000 appropriately chose HIV/AIDS, under the formal conference title "HIV/AIDS: The Greatest Leadership Challenge."

It turned out to be like so many conferences designed and driven by the United Nations: a marathon talk-fest, with a program of action or declaration at the end. Mind you, to be fair (an instinct of which I am not enamoured), there was also a great deal of networking amongst the delegates which can serve usefully for the future.

But hidden in the media entrails of this gathering was an announcement that was of immense significance. It held the prospect of dramatically changing life for vast numbers of children in Africa.

Carol Bellamy, at that time right at the midpoint of her tenure as executive director of UNICEF and at the absolute height of her power, held a press conference to announce that UNICEF would initiate a campaign to abolish school fees across the continent. The decision to hold the press conference was well-considered: Carol was responding to the urgent entreaties of UNICEF's staff on the ground in

Africa, who doubtless understood the situation better than anyone else.

The press release is worth quoting directly:

> In a bold initiative to put education at the forefront of the fight against HIV/AIDS, UNICEF Executive Director Carol Bellamy today called on African leaders to join a campaign to abolish all education fees and other costs for primary school-age children . . . "We live in a world where children whose families cannot pay for tuition, uniforms, desks, pencils, books and building repairs are shut out of classrooms," Bellamy said . . . "Placing every child in a classroom has never been more urgent than it is today. Under threat from the pandemic, children must be able to turn to schools as places of learning, inclusion, stability and life-saving information about HIV/AIDS. No child should be barred entry . . . Governments have both a legal and a moral responsibility to fulfill that obligation," she stressed.

It was a truly important, and unexpected, promulgation.

It's worth remembering that when, at the UN Millennium General Assembly of 2000, the countries of the world convened to establish the Millennium Development Goals, or "MDGS," they unreservedly included, as one of the goals, universal access to primary education. In so doing, they were reaffirming Article 28, sub-1(a) of the Convention on the Rights of the Child: "Make primary education compulsory and available free to all . . ." The numbers of children excluded range somewhere between

105 and 120 million worldwide, 44 million in Africa, about 60 percent of them girls.

Now no one should think that this is anything new. On twenty-one different occasions over the last seventy years, dating back to the International Conference on Education in 1934, the international community has endorsed primary school education as a human right of every child everywhere, and argued that every single child must be in school. The reasons are well-known: everyone agrees that primary education is the salvation of struggling societies, that every additional year of schooling — beyond providing the glorious wellspring of knowledge — brings with it the best chance to defeat poverty, the best chance for better parenting, better health, better nutrition, greater opportunity, and a direct line to economic growth. From UNESCO to UNICEF to the World Bank, it is agreed that universal primary education is the ultimate vector of human progress.

So it is that alongside the MDGS, at least five other international declarations drawn up since 2000 have committed governments, north and south, to placing every child in school. There's probably no other international norm so fully, repeatedly, and universally embraced.

How then is it possible that the burden of school fees in Africa bedevils school attendance to this day? Even where governments introduce the abolition of fees, there always seems to be some compromising twist in the formula, so that the abolition is never fully complete. Either books or uniforms are excluded (and they can be costly), or the individual schools tack on "registration fees," or "examination fees," or "parent-teacher fees," which make attendance for many children impossible.

The words of the executive director of UNICEF, therefore, were of signal significance. They meant that the world's premier children's agency would throw its weight behind a cancellation campaign, the result of which would surely be the emancipation of huge numbers of children, otherwise excluded from schooling. This was especially crucial for children orphaned by AIDS who lived in abject poverty, with no prospect of having the resources to pay for school.

Except that nothing happened! Nothing. Having stoked the fires of expectation, UNICEF then abdicated responsibility. It was shocking. Only now, almost five years later, has UNICEF shown an active interest again.

What went wrong? How can it be explained?

It would seem that when Carol Bellamy returned to New York, her headquarters staff pounced on her, and urged her to reconsider. The arguments, I believe, were several in number: UNICEF was about to sponsor a UN Special Session on children, originally scheduled for September of 2001 (as it turned out, postponed to May of 2002 because of 9/11), and it was felt by her inspired intelligentsia that some countries might be offended by the initiative on school fees; her imaginative education division was paralyzed by the thought of school overcrowding and the availability of teachers if large numbers of children descended on the schools; her financial strategists felt that the resources were not in place to provide compensatory funding to governments that took the abolition plunge. Overall, the mood of the resident visionaries was almost Pavlovian in its opposition. The idea was dropped.

I could speak about the poverty of imagination, but that seems inadequate somehow. The dramatic shift in position constituted a retreat from UNICEF's mandate. The Convention on the Rights of the Child, which is effectively UNICEF's mission statement, couldn't be clearer. The Millennium Development Goal couldn't be clearer. Carol Bellamy's position in Addis Ababa couldn't be clearer. This was not some negotiable item. I'm writing and speaking passionately about it because, every time I travel to Africa, I encounter orphan children who are desperate to be in school, who need friends and teachers and attention, who need one meal a day that could come from a school feeding program, who need the sense of self-worth that education could bring, who want so much to learn, and who are denied all of it because the costs of schooling are prohibitive.

The yearning within every child to be in school is a viscerally powerful instinct. I well remember working on a UN study in the mid-1990s titled "The Impact of Armed Conflict on Children." The expert for the study was Graça Machel, former minister of education in Mozambique, appointed by the Secretary-General because of her unrivalled commitment to Africa's children, stemming in part from the desolate situation of children in Mozambique after the fratricidal civil war. Graça travelled all over the world during the two years of the study, observing and documenting the state of children in war zones from the

Middle East to Colombia, from Sri Lanka to Burundi. When she came to draft her recommendations, it was fascinating to see that the first substantive item on her list was to get every child into school, whether during conflict or after conflict — not just because she thought it best, but because the children wanted it, wanted it more than anything else.

I remember so well speaking to children who had been through the genocide in Rwanda, speaking to children physically and emotionally scarred by the conflict in northern Uganda, speaking to children orphaned by AIDS, and when asked the question, "How can I be of help to you . . . what do you most want?" they would all answer in identical terms, "I want to go to school."

We lost five years of potential school for millions of kids because of the hiatus between the promise of 2000 and the promise of restored impetus today. It's like so much of internationalism: no one pays attention, the media are uncritical, the commitments and obligations are expendable, the organizations, expected to perform, don't perform and yet emerge unscathed. They're almost never called to account.

Ah, you might say, but surely these agencies have governing bodies of UN member states that oversee policies made by the secretariats and can intervene where necessary. Yes, that's absolutely true. But the sorry reality about the UNICEF executive board that I observed in the four years that I attended board meetings was its essential impotence. (I attended all board meetings as one of Carol's two deputies, in my case the deputy executive director responsible for overall UNICEF programming and external relations.) There are thirty-eight countries on the UNICEF board, represented, as often as not, by junior diplomats (junior in status if not in age) who don't know what questions to ask, or what challenges to pose, or what speeches to make. They're preposterously deferential and uncritical. Occasionally, to be sure, you get a cantankerous diplomat who confronts the secretariat, but the secretariat finesses issues with the ease of an accomplished artisan in the local workshop of smoke and mirrors. Many's the time I wanted, with subversive intent, to plant a question or two, just to have real issues actually discussed. But I couldn't bring myself to do it; it was too risky. The whole point was to end these nuisance board meetings as quickly as possible (during Carol's tenure, we almost always ended at least half a day early); it would have caused a form of rabid consternation were things prolonged. Somebody would have smelled a rat if an informed or probing question was asked, and a witch-hunt would have followed. I could practically see myself hanging beside the flags outside the UN building on First Avenue.

It would never happen that someone on the board would say to Carol Bellamy, or to one of her deputies, "What about that campaign against school fees? Was it real? Was it just a grand gesture that had no hope of implementation? Do you not think it rash to call for a campaign leading down a garden path, where the path is strewn with the hopes of children whose rights you are pledged to protect?" To suggest the possibility of posing such questions is to induce laughter.

And if I may digress for one moment further, the response of Carol's staff to the question of school fees illuminates a congenital timidity within the UN system. Time and time again, staff at agencies and at the central secretariat conjure up visions of conflict with member states, should the staff ever take unusual or controversial initiatives. That may be true when dealing with matters of peace and security (Iraq, Darfur, the Middle East, suicide bombers), but it's not true for interventions that are fundamentally humanitarian in nature — particularly those already defended in a convention ratified by every member state, save two. Member governments can almost always be won over or influenced or shamed; it's just that the atmosphere within the UN family is often so clutched, so neurotically tentative, that no one wants to take the chance.

And that, I believe, is what happened with school fees. It became more important to appease some imaginary opposition, or to balk at the challenge of overcoming obstacles, than to address the desperate needs of children. This state of pusillanimity wasn't helped by the fact that school fees emanated from structural adjustment policies fashioned by the World Bank, and no one wanted to lock horns with the Bank.

Don't misunderstand me. I know that this is strong stuff, but in personal terms, I loved my work with UNICEF, and I loved collaborating with so many talented colleagues, especially staff in the middle ranks. I think the agency has more potential than any other organization within the United Nations family. That's why it drives me crazy when UNICEF opts out of the job it is mandated to perform.

The capacity of UNICEF to turn the world around was demonstrated in the years of James Grant, the executive director who preceded Carol Bellamy. For fifteen years, from 1980 to 1995, Jim Grant, liberal democrat, passionate idealist, brilliant tactician, showed the world an astonishing level of accomplishment, and is reckoned to have saved the lives of twenty-five million children over that period. How did he do it? Precisely by setting measurable goals and targets, and then rallying the entire organization, and governments, and civil society, and political will to achieve the seemingly impossible. It was Jim and UNICEF who fashioned the Child Survival Revolution incorporating, amongst other initiatives, universal child immunization against six preventable diseases; breastfeeding; oral rehydration therapy to prevent death from dehydration; mass distribution of vitamin A to put a brake on malnutrition, death, and blindness; and then on to iodizing salt so that hundreds of thousands of children were spared severe retardation. He travelled relentlessly, crazily, indefatigably, from developing country to developing country, always with a sachet of oral rehydration salts in his pocket to be pulled out at every state banquet for a public discussion, over foie gras, of diarrhea, without the slightest twitch of embarrassment. He understood, as no one had understood before him, that the galvanizing of political leadership and the mobilization of entire societies could rout the demons of childhood illness.

He succeeded to a remarkable extent. In all my twenty-one years in the orbit of the United Nations, I have never seen anyone approximate the feats of Jim Grant. What was it that Mark Antony said of Caesar, "When comes such another?" The answer is, never. If Jim Grant had announced the abolishment of school fees, then by this time there wouldn't be a country left that dared to maintain fees, and if his staff had given him a hard time, his eyes would have glittered with the challenge of proving them wrong. It isn't that he wouldn't brook opposition; it's simply that he swept opposition into the roiling tides of success. In this instance, it would be millions of children in school today who are not in school.

You might well ask, then, why didn't he undertake a campaign to abolish fees? Remember the timing: Jim Grant had been executive director of UNICEF for ten years before the Convention on the Rights of the Child became binding international law, with its provision on universal, free, and compulsory primary education. He was at the time — 1990 — leading the Child Survival Revolution, attempting to do what no one had done before: to dramatically lower the toll of fourteen million deaths every year in the under-five age group. Predictably, that objective consumed the energies of Grant and the entire organization. As Hillary Rodham Clinton said at Jim's funeral, "he saved more lives — twenty-five million — in the past fifteen years than any other person in the world." What's more, before he died, in January of 1995, he laid the groundwork to implement the full Convention on the

Rights of the Child, including cancellation of school fees. It was up to his successor to finish the job. It didn't happen.

On the other hand, in the grand scheme of things, I cannot take myself off the hook. During the last half of the nineties, it became more and more evident that the AIDS virus was eating away at the development gains we might otherwise have achieved. It was difficult to reduce maternal mortality when death stalked the women of the continent. It was impossible to reduce child mortality when the combination of poverty, malnutrition, and AIDS was decimating infant life. I, personally, as someone responsible for overall country programming, should have been ringing alarm bells earlier. I failed to do so, and I'm culpable, and I'm not going to try to hide it. But at least, by the time I left UNICEF in early November 1999, I had fully grasped what was happening on AIDS, and was determined to devote myself to doing something about it. Indeed, the whole world began to take notice: it was in January 2000 that the Security Council met to discuss HIV/AIDS, the first time in its history that it convened to address an issue of health.

But let me back up slightly to relate a sequence of events which speaks directly to primary education and ties everything together.

In the fall of 1999, just before I left UNICEF, Carol Bellamy prevailed on me to go to Johannesburg to meet with Nelson Mandela and Graça Machel, to attempt to persuade them to provide the personal leadership for a UNICEF-driven initiative that would come to be known as the Global Movement for Children. The idea was in its earliest stages, gradually being defined, but the principle was to mobilize African leaders in advance of the second Summit for Children, to be held in September of 2001. The three putative themes were education, HIV/AIDS, and armed conflict.

Graça Machel was a close personal friend, and she was and is always willing to arrange a homey gathering with Madiba (Mandela's colloquial name) if circumstances permit. Circumstances did permit, and one warm, quiet day in September, we gathered in their dining room for lunch and conversation. It was a fascinating, if unsettling experience. After I'd set out the general idea of the initiative, and the potential subject matters, Mandela cross-examined me with penetrating intensity. What exactly would it mean; what would be asked of them; what support would be provided; would their involvement be substantive, or was it merely an exercise in public relations? I answered as best I could by the seat of my rhetorical pants. He was clearly skeptical. Time and time again, Madiba was asked to participate in well-intentioned causes, meetings, activities, and he had learned, through painful experience, to approach all invitations with caution. It was a question of divining which causes were real, and which were window-dressing. I think both Graça and Madiba felt that if this invitation was so important, why hadn't Carol Bellamy come herself?

In any event, after an exchange of roughly half an hour, Madiba scrutinized me closely, heaved a weary sigh, and agreed to participate. He was, nonetheless, still reluctant, and as it turned out, his reluctance had a touch of clairvoyance.

What happened next was disheartening. Upon my return from South Africa, I had written a quite excited memo about the willingness of Graça and Madiba to be involved; it was practically my last act in UNICEF. I then departed from the agency, only to learn, months later, that my departure was followed by virtual silence where Graça and Madiba were concerned. There was absolutely no significant follow-up from the UNICEF side for several months. It was as if our meeting had been purely ephemeral.

I must admit that I was acutely embarrassed, and appealed to UNICEF to make contact. Finally, well into the year 2000, UNICEF got back in touch with the Machel-Mandela duo. This in turn led to many lengthy palavers, over many months' duration, about what, exactly, to do next. Eventually, Graça and Madiba agreed to attend the summit themselves, and to lobby African leaders to do the same in the hope of moving the agenda for children forward dramatically. As mentioned earlier, the summit dates were then shifted to May 2002 because of 9/11.

By the time we had entered 2002, children orphaned by AIDS had begun to overwhelm African countries, and it was felt that in addition to the summit, the key players had best be brought together at some separate point during the year to confront the escalating crisis. I was by then firmly in the envoy role, and again Carol asked me to try to persuade Madiba and Graça to effectively "host" a meeting on orphans in Johannesburg in the fall.

So Madiba, Graça, and I had another lunch, this time in New York during the Special Session in May 2002. We were joined by two other good friends and colleagues, Anurita Bains and Theo Sowa, who were working closely with Graça on the issues affecting African children. I remember the lunch well because I became exceedingly emotional in talking about the orphans, and I suspect that Graça and Madiba agreed to consider seriously the proposed future meeting partly to relieve us all of the embarrassment that flowed from my somewhat extravagant loss of self-control.

In any event, they came on board, and the meeting was convened in September 2002. It was, in its own way, an unusual gathering, one long day in duration. Nelson Mandela opened the proceedings with a stirring and heartfelt address. He then stayed through a brilliant overview presentation provided by Alan Whiteside, the professorial guru on AIDS from the University of Natal. Graça Machel remained the entire day and participated extensively. Carol Bellamy attended from beginning to end, and the rest of the participants, numbering roughly forty-five, represented international NGOs, such as Save the Children and CARE, through to indigenous African activists from Sibongile Mkhabela, the CEO of the Nelson Mandela Children's Fund, to Angélique Kidjo, the magnificent singer from Benin. Staff from UNICEF and UNAIDS were there in profusion.

There were plenaries and there were break-out sessions. The conversations were heated, creative, and inspired. Every group was charged with fashioning an agenda of intervention. Every group answered the challenge.

It was my job to wind up the conference and to set out the essence of the agenda. The number-one item I dealt with, the item on which there was unanimous agreement, the item about which there was the greatest sense of urgency was, predictably, the elimination of school fees! Thus do things come full circle.

The issue of school fees continued to surface repetitively. The meeting in Jo'burg in 2002 was followed the next year by a similar — indeed, expanded — meeting in Geneva, with exactly the same singular recommendation. It's not that there weren't a thousand other things that the assembled multilateral and NGO experts suggested to ease life for orphan children; it's just that the abolition of school fees always rose to the head of the class. These annual speakathons soon had a name, the Global Partners Forum, and while I have a genuine respect for the roll call of participants, the partners forums, from the outset, gave credence to the proposition that if you talk about something for long enough, the illusion will be created that progress is being made. And I suppose there has been some progress in the world of reports, analyses, figures, tables, diagrams, and at least a thousand PowerPoint presentations, not to overlook throbbing intellectual rumination, but very little progress that's discernible in the lives of orphaned and vulnerable children on the ground.

Just like the eradication of poverty, the commitment to gender equity, and the struggle against the pandemic, the truth is that free primary education, thus far at least, is all talk and endless negotiation. The commitments made are commitments dashed.

I often wonder, in an increasingly jaded way, how long the children of Africa will have to wait before the world delivers. You can't begin to imagine the numbers of reports that have been produced demonstrating the needs of orphan children and demanding the abolition of school fees. They proliferate in unimaginable numbers. It's almost a travesty — no, not almost; it is a travesty — the way in which document after document pours off the presses, especially the multilateral presses, making the same points ad nauseam unto eternity, containing the same figures, positing the same recommendations. In fact, an argument can plausibly be made that the reports have become a kind of Machiavellian delaying tactic. You want action? Wait — there's something else to read.

And inevitably, it never stops. Just take a look at 2005:

When the Millennium Development report was published in January 2005, Jeffrey Sachs, economist and primary author, called for an end to school fees. In fact, he went so far as to include it at the top of his list of Quick Wins. When the Secretary-General responded to that report, setting out his agenda for the grand debate on the MDGs in the General Assembly in September, he included the need to eliminate school fees. When Prime Minister Tony Blair launched his Commission for Africa report in March, the abolition of school fees occupied a place of pride amongst the recommendations. When the African Union met in June to discuss matters of educational policy, the abolition of school fees figured prominently in the preparatory papers.

After all, it makes such powerful sense. Let me elaborate: The impulse towards abolition started with Malawi. Between 1995 and 2000, Malawi was joined by Uganda, Lesotho, and Tanzania (Lesotho, interestingly, has introduced it one grade per year). Between 2001 and 2005, Mozambique, Zambia, Madagascar, Kenya, Benin, Cameroon, and Ghana came on board. Some of these countries have had startling results. When Malawi eliminated school fees, enrolment increased by more than 50 percent. In the case of Uganda, enrolment went up by nearly 70 percent, from 3.4 to 5.7 million students.

By extraordinary coincidence, I was present when President Museveni decided to lift Uganda's fees. It was after a conference on education in Kampala, in March 1996. (I remember it well, because a group of young girls performed a stirring piece of theatre depicting the way they were sexually harassed and assaulted by boys on the way to and from school, and by teachers at school.) The UNICEF head of office, the representative, had been pressing Museveni to do away with school fees. We sat with the president in an ante chamber of the conference centre, with his minister of gender and the minister of education. Museveni abruptly said he intended to lift the fees for primary school for four children in every family (an election campaign was looming). The UNICEF representative made an impassioned case that, wherever possible, two of the four children should be girls. With an impatient smile on his face, the president agreed. Thus is policy made: a spontaneous idea happens to be expressed to the right person at the right time, and presto, without so much as a murmur of hesitation, millions of lives are changed.

In 1999, when Cameroon eliminated school fees, the primary gross enrolment rate went up some 15 percent. But Tanzania topped them all: when it abolished fees in 2001, the numbers went up 100 percent, from 1.5 to 3 million students in one year. President Mkapa had this to say in an article in the *International Herald Tribune,* in July 2004, commenting on the relationship between debt reduction and the immediate value for education in particular: "We abolished school fees in primary schools . . . Gender parity has been attained . . . 31,825 classrooms and 7,530 teachers houses have been constructed . . . 17,851 new teachers have been recruited and 14,852 have been sent to upgrading courses . . . the pass rate in primary school has risen from 19 percent in 1999 to 40 percent in 2003; some 12,689 school committees have been trained to build capacity . . ."

That's a particularly satisfying piece of modern history, because two wrongs were righted: Tanzania was relieved of its debt, and the country could afford once again to educate its children. Naturally, it wasn't the cancellation of debts alone; there was also assistance from donors and a significant re-allocation within the government's budget. But it shows what can be done. As President Mkapa said, "I have written this article to show that it is indeed possible to achieve the Millennium Development Goal targets if we are all committed to putting the right pillars in place."

The most dramatic recent expression of the episodic return-to-school policy (or perhaps it should be called the start-school policy) was the case of Kenya. In the election at the end of 2002, the leading presidential contender, Mwai Kibaki, promised an end to school fees. The country exploded with joy. No other election promise came close to competing with the abolition of school fees, and rather more important, once elected, President Kibaki did exactly as he said: the fees were lifted.

Little more than a month later, in January 2003, one million, three hundred thousand Kenyan children who had not been in school before turned up at the doors of the schools. It was, in every way, sensational; enrolment leaped from 5.9 to 7.2 million children. Inevitably, a significant percentage of the new recruits were children orphaned by AIDS.

On the face of it, therefore, there is real momentum established for the abolition of fees. But as much as that is true, it's important not to get carried away. It would seem that even when tuition fees are abolished, there are so many other costs — books, compulsory uniforms, fees for registration, for parent-teacher associations, for community associations, or to write examinations — that active vigilance is still required. What we are after is universal, unimpeded, unequivocal free education — absolutely no costs, hidden or otherwise. That's what it says in the Convention on the Rights of the Child; that's what the international community, in theory at least, has agreed to. So while I'm happy to enumerate the success stories, there are sobering caveats.

Note that when the World Bank did a worldwide survey in 2005, seventy-six of ninety-two developing countries canvassed still had some form of user fees acting as deterrents to attendance. One way or the other, families living on less than a dollar a day simply can't afford to pay a tithe for their children to go to school.

The issue is further muddled by the professional Cassandras, doomsayers, and general members of the "share no joy" society. Their strident voices are prophets of cataclysm, warning that schools will collapse under the weight of new pupils, teachers can't handle astronomically enlarged classes, and ministries of education have made no plans to address the financial consequences. Those assumptions are not without a touch of validity. For example, in the case of Malawi, the cancellation of fees was admirably spontaneous, but without any advance planning. As a result, the country found itself short by thirteen thousand teachers and thirty-eight thousand classrooms. Worse, for various political reasons, there was only marginal external support and the resources, early on, failed to materialize. The educational consequences were sad: of the 1.3 million students who entered grade one in 1994, only three hundred thousand made it to the end of the educational cycle in 2002.

But it doesn't have to be that way. Uganda has had the opposite experience simply by careful planning. Even Malawi is now in control of its educational destiny, having made the predictable mid-course correction. When all is said and done, it's better to scramble somewhat in the aftermath (exactly what Kenya is now doing to good purpose) than to continue to exclude children from school on the destructive basis of class and income. Kenya reallocated $60 million from other sectors, then the World Bank chimed in with $50 million, the U.K. development arm provided $6 million, and UNICEF contributed $2.5 million. All is not perfect, but the world has changed for the children of Kenya now that the fees are gone.

In a recent UNESCO newsletter, the then assistant director general for education, John Daniel (now president and CEO of the Commonwealth of Learning based in Vancouver) wrote, "UNESCO believes that it is better to uphold the principle of free primary education, and to address energetically the quality challenge posed by an enrolment surge, than to ration access to school through fees."

Nicely put. Very nicely put.

It's so interesting, and such a poignant commentary on the resolve of the international community, that we are unable to put every child into school when we're all of a mind that nothing is more important to a child's present and future. In fact, as others have observed, it's fundamental to a child's life or death. I recently saw the printout of a PowerPoint presentation made by Donald Bundy of the World Bank's Human Development Network. One of the slides was stunning. It reviewed the HIV prevalence rates, by educational levels, in rural Uganda from 1990 to 2001 for individuals between the ages of eighteen and twenty-nine. In 2001, those with secondary education had a prevalence rate of under 2 percent; those with primary education had a prevalence rate just over

6 percent; those with no formal education had a prevalence rate just over 12 percent.

Is that not sufficient, in and of itself, to make the case for free and universal primary education?

We've been wrestling with it for so long.

It was back in Jomtien, Thailand, in 1990, when a major international conference, attracting eighty-seven countries, hatched the slogan "Education for All by the year 2000" (or EFA, as it came to be known). The year 1990 had special significance: in September, the first-ever Summit for Children, under the auspices of UNICEF, was held in New York, and barely two months later, the Convention on the Rights of the Child had received the necessary twenty ratifications to be considered an instrument of binding international law. The world thought that educational policies would finally move forward for children: the stars were in alignment.

The world was wrong. Maybe we all should have thought back to Alma-Ata in 1978, when an analogous conference had coined the phrase "Health for All by the year 2000," only to see those hopes irrevocably dashed. When the international community gathered in Amman, Jordan, in 1995, to assess progress since the education conference in Jomtien, the findings were, as always, painfully incremental. I actually attended that meeting and can vouch for the rhetorical flim-flam which attempted to make a cashmere throw out of a newt's tongue, but it didn't work. No one was buying. So, admirable punching bags for punishment that countries are, they all met again in Dakar, Senegal, in 2000, and resolved to achieve what they had promised to achieve ten years earlier.

Universal primary education has remained as elusive as ever. The fact is that school enrolment rates now are roughly where they were a quarter century ago. Indeed, rates in twenty-seven countries have declined over the last five to ten years, and the World Bank estimates that eighty-eight countries will not meet the MDG of universal primary education by 2015.

Little wonder, given the pace of what is termed progress.

For me, the most stunning evidence of a complete lack of urgency — not to mention a curious lapse of memory — on the part of the international community came at a "sub-meeting," co-sponsored by the World Bank and UNICEF in mid-December of 2004. Almost exactly four years to the day after the famous (infamous) press conference at the African Development Forum in Addis, Carol Bellamy, in her opening remarks, again — without so much as the faintest tint of cheek-reddening — proclaimed the crucial need to abolish school fees. And then came Jim Wolfensohn, president of the World Bank, who emphasized exactly the same priority, adding the astonishingly disingenuous observation that he wasn't sure if school fees were a feature of World Bank Structural Adjustment Programs, but if they were, that era was well past, and the time to act was now.

Again, an aside. I well remember that when I worked at UNICEF in the late nineties, the head of the education section was a woman named Fay Chung. As it happened,

Fay Chung was Zimbabwean, and the minister of education in the Mugabe government at the very time that Zimbabwe introduced "cost-sharing," (i.e., school fees). She vividly recollected school fees as part of the web of conditionality imposed by the World Bank in return for a loan. But that's not all. Shortly after Kenya abolished school fees, effective in January 2003, I met with the minister of education in his office in Nairobi to discuss how the government had managed it, particularly the financing. He said — I was taken by surprise — that he had been minister of finance in a prior government of Kenya when, in return for a World Bank loan, school fees were introduced. He was therefore entirely comfortable in demanding that the Bank help with compensatory financing when school fees were abolished, having done the damage in the first place.

In that same article in the UNESCO newsletter quoted earlier, entitled "The price of school fees," there appears the following: "Even the World Bank has joined the bandwagon, by making a 160 degree turn in policy and encouraging countries to remove school fees. Who can forget the mantra of 'cost recovery' which the Bank began hammering in the late 1980s . . ."

It is beyond me how anyone can pretend that the World Bank and the IMF weren't involved in a destructive pattern of user fees, imposed throughout the eighties and nineties.

The most interesting aspect about Wolfensohn's speech, however, was the lugubrious tone in which he cast the latest omnibus education scheme for developing countries. It's called the Fast-Track Initiative (FTI), and it seeks to provide universal basic education by having the donor governments contribute a minimum of $4 billion a year for several years. The promise to do so was made at the meeting in Dakar in 2000, and so far, said Wolfensohn, in a tone of derisive resignation, the Bank, which effectively runs FTI, has received $300 million. It gives new definition to the word "shortfall."

But what makes it all the more distressing is the present preoccupation with this so-called Fast-Track Initiative, allegedly designed to provide the educational panacea that has eluded the world for so long. It is promoted as the promised land for education.

But it won't work. It's fundamentally flawed in too many ways.

In saying that, I realize that I'm on a sticky wicket. The FTI is supported by a large number of NGOs, working together in what is called the Global Campaign for Education. They see the FTI as the only viable initiative presently in play. And because it's the only initiative in play, they're willing to choke back their reservations, even expressing them publicly on occasion, but ultimately embracing the FTI, believing, in an almost touching display of political innocence, that it can be rescued from within.

It's notable that the same people who will go to the barricades for debt, trade, and aid, are willing to compromise on education. And so, though it pains me more than I can say, I must take issue with friends and activists in civil society.

The FTI is based on two significant premises: First, that the country seeking endorsement by the initiative has what is called a Poverty Reduction Strategy Paper as the basis for country-wide socio-economic policy; second, that it has a credible education-sector plan. Immediately, there are problems. The Poverty Reduction Strategies are the contemporary metamorphosis, the latest incarnation, of the old structural adjustment ideology, a not-so-skilful manipulation of the most offensive aspects of structural adjustment in order to make the new financial regimen acceptable to the developing country. What was supposed to make them palatable was the fact that civil society would be fully involved in the Poverty Reduction Strategy Papers' formulation.

It has not happened. The participation of civil society has ranged from trivial to marginal. Basically the Poverty Reduction Strategies haven't worked, although they're sustained by a propaganda machine of impressive proportions. Whenever any of us have been critical, there's been quite a heated response, in part because the International Financial Institutions, having lost credibility over structural adjustment, are darned if they're going to let it happen again.

But they failed to anticipate attacks from two entirely unexpected quarters. In May of 2005, the United Nations Development Programme released a new report with the impossibly clunky title, "MDG-based Poverty Reduction Strategy Papers need more ambitious economic policies." What it argued, in a nutshell, was that reaching the Millennium Development Goals requires the abandonment of the antediluvian macroeconomic conditions imposed on poor developing countries. This was no small matter: it's almost unheard of that a UN agency should disparage the orthodoxy of the World Bank and the IMF. It speaks to the growing awareness that civil society has not really been consulted in the design of Poverty Reduction Strategy Papers, and that the International Financial Institutions are behaving with unlovely arrogance.

More specifically, the UNDP challenged overall Poverty Reduction Strategy policies on four grounds: First, that they give priority to satisfying the World Bank and the IMF and the donors, rather than the developing country; second, that they pay far too little attention to job creation and the need for increased incomes to alleviate poverty; third, that they depreciate the value of public investment; and fourth, that they support privatization of public services like water and electricity, which support has a record so mixed as to jeopardize the attainment of the MDGS.

That's pretty tough stuff, all in all.

But there's more, because the UNDP report was preceded in March of 2005 by yet another document of surprising dissent from the normal international financial prescriptions. It was issued as a United Kingdom policy paper by Hilary Benn, the secretary of state for international development, entitled "Partnerships for Poverty Reduction: Rethinking Conditionality." It was a pretty frontal assault on the way the International Financial Institutions order the world, and the way in which they continue to impose conditionality even as they pretend the opposite. The flavour of the argument is easily captured in Hilary Benn's foreword: "Development cannot be imposed. It can only be facilitated. It requires ownership, participation and empowerment, not harangues and dictates."

The document is so sensible, so restrained, and yet so damning that I shall simply quote a few brief extracts:

> We will not make our aid conditional on specific policy decisions by partner governments, or attempt to impose policy choices on them (including in sensitive economic areas such as privatization or trade liberalization). . . .
>
> We believe that it is inappropriate and has proven to be ineffective for donors to impose policies on developing countries. . . .
>
> The U.K. Government accepts the evidence that conditionality cannot "buy" policy change which countries do not want. . . .
>
> Questions remain about the amount of genuine autonomy enjoyed by (developing) countries, given the greater financial power and technical capacity of donors . . .

Taken together, the UNDP and U.K. government papers constitute an indictment of the way things are currently done.

And I'd expand on the indictment from my own personal experience in the field. It's just not appropriate to be giving so much power and authority to the donors holding posts in the various countries. The donor diplomats vary wildly in competence and involvement. The tendency is for the most voluble or the most laden with disposable currency to lead the way for everyone else. Their judgement can be way off, their prejudices worn on their sleeves. I can't tell you how many meetings of donors I've attended at which their views of the national administration bordered on slander, so intensely colonial it could turn your stomach. That's not true of all, of course: there were some thoroughly committed diplomats. But there were far too many who resented their posting to a minor African country, and glowered their way through every meeting. What's more, a surprising number of western diplomats had seldom ventured beyond the capitals; they lived lives of rumour informed by gossip. It always left a sour taste in my mouth. And they were so stubbornly opinionated, so omniscient. And often so wrong. I'm afraid that my encounters were sometimes unpleasant because it was difficult to maintain silence in the face of mindless and unwarranted views.

I remember one instance, in Lesotho, where the ambassadorial crew locked horns with the Ministry of Health over voluntary and confidential counselling and testing (VCT) for HIV/AIDS. The ministry wanted to open VCT centres across the country (an approach common to nearly all countries), but the foreign diplomats had decided that there were not enough counsellors, and they fought the intended policy every step of the way. I was in on one of those meetings; it was tense, angry and unproductive. The government felt compromised because the donors held the purse strings. The donors felt empowered because they held the purse strings. As it happens, the donors couldn't have been more wrong, nor the government more right. In the end, the Ministry of Health carried the day, but you have to ask yourself how the donors had the presumption to decide that they, and not the government, would determine public policy.

I remember witnessing a similar incident in Malawi. The government wanted to proceed with treatment as quickly as possible. The diplomatic community railed against the idea, insisting that there was neither enough money nor enough human capacity to make any significant advance. But the government's determination derived from an assessment made by three visiting experts from the World Health Organization (WHO), who were persuaded that with the hiring of a handful of additional people, Malawi could begin a significant treatment initiative; indeed, they thought that Malawi would be in a position to put fifty thousand people into treatment fairly speedily. In the nastiest fashion, the bilateral diplomats cast sneering aspersion on the WHO experts and fought the government plans. The government persisted, and in the figures released by the WHO in June 2005, Malawi had between eighteen thousand and twenty-three thousand people receiving antiretroviral drugs, representing between 11 and 14 percent of those who qualified for treatment. That may seem low, but in percentage terms it's higher than Mozambique, Tanzania, Ethiopia, South Africa, Zimbabwe, Ghana, or Nigeria.

Thus, the diplomats were wrong again.

Allow me, then, to return to education, and to the unacceptable reliance on the Poverty Reduction Strategy Papers as the basis for the Fast-Track Initiative. If the Poverty Reduction Strategies are found wanting, as they have been found wanting, then what point to embed educational reform in their tattered intellectual and financial rationales? No point, I would argue.

Pared down to its basics, the FTI works this way: The education plan of each country is measured against the FTI's guidelines (read: conditions), and then requires endorsement from the donor in-country team. If that endorsement is given, the plan then goes to the FTI steering committee in Washington, which makes the final decision about whether or not the plan is eligible for funding. If a plan were to be submitted at the time of this writing, the steering committee would consist of the United Kingdom, Sweden, the United States, the World Bank, and UNESCO. Who, you might well ask, represents the interests of the applicant country?

Frankly it's offensive, and I don't intend to beat around the bush. It's the latest form of neo-colonial chic, and it has no place in progressive development programming in the modern world. It divides countries into supplicants and benefactors, on the flawed assumption that somehow the benefactors care about education. If they did, we wouldn't be in this jackpot: according to the Global Campaign for Education, there is a financing gap of $5.5 billion a year. What right have the gap-ists to dictate terms?

In fact, the Global Campaign for Education is well aware of the FTI's flaws. Recently they released their own critique of the FTI with the provocative title, "Small Change: An alternative progress report on the education Fast-Track Initiative." They talk about the FTI as "beginning to look like a global scam for *avoiding* the Monterrey and Dakar commitments" and go on to say, "The FTI is perceived in many quarters as a 'donor-driven' initiative. Some fundamental changes to its decision-making structures and processes are needed . . . Both developing country governments and civil society need to be formally represented in FTI governance structures. Their lack of power and influence . . . has not only undermined ownership at the global level, but may also weaken the country assessment and reform process."

"A scam," "donor-driven," "fundamental changes," "lack of power and influence"? How does the Global Campaign for Education justify its support? One of the coalition's members, the British NGO ActionAid, released a separate critique, equally scathing. They faulted the FTI on several grounds, allowing them to conclude, "The report finds that without important changes, the Fast-Track will have only a limited impact on the challenge of achieving the 2015 goal of universal basic education."

I don't get it. Rarely have I seen support vacillate so wildly from lukewarm to hypothermia. And of course the Global Campaign folk are right to vibrate with ambivalence. The FTI has no evident redeeming features: it's run by the donors; it's fraught with ill-concealed conditionality; it's based on increasingly discredited Poverty

Reduction Strategy Papers; it confers the possibility of free primary education only on those developing countries with harmonious donor relations; and it's focused so obsessively on dollars as to miss the prospect of creating a school system that is the centrepiece of every community. I suppose you could swallow some of it if the money was flowing, but the money is trickling in droplets.

And I haven't even touched on the weaknesses of the actual FTI guidelines. Suffice to say they're lousy on gender, they're reactionary on teachers' salaries and salary caps, they're confused on student grade repetition rates, they're out to lunch on the impact of AIDS, and the entire venture does little for the poor, for civil society, or for the indispensable role of the school in the life of the child.

I don't think the FTI can be rehabilitated from the inside or the outside. It should be scrapped. UNICEF should intervene and reclaim the educational domain. (Certainly UNESCO has neither the resources nor the staff on the ground to play the central role. In fact, for many, when free primary education and UNESCO are mentioned in the same breath, eyes turn heavenwards.) What we need is a new approach, country by country, where the country makes the decisions, designs the interventions and abolishes school fees of every kind, and UNICEF provides expert technical assistance on the one hand, and organizes the collective financial international response on the other — a perfect test of the stated intentions of the G8.

It would be great penance for UNICEF, and if they unleashed half the zeal of a Jim Grant, every eligible child would be in school before 2015. Instead of looking down the maw of eternity, children would see an immediate future. Just imagine: a crucial MDG would be fulfilled. I don't even think it would be that tough. One of the reasons the resources are so scarce is the sense of disarray and skepticism that attaches to the FTI.

Where education is concerned, the IFIs have a debt of their own to pay back to Africa. The World Bank and the International Monetary Fund should foot the bill for free primary education. In other circumstances, it would be called reparations; in present circumstances, it should be called mandatory restitution.

We're really in a desperate race against time here. That fact is driven home to me in every trip I make to Africa. During my most recent visit to western Kenya, in July 2005, I met with the principal of a primary school of 500 students. Incredibly enough, 230 are orphans, the great majority orphaned by AIDS. The looming question, raised with me repeatedly, is: What happens to these impoverished kids after primary school? Are their educational lives terminated? Secondary school costs a lot, everywhere. No country has free secondary education.

In this local instance in Kenya, special circumstances allow for five scholarships for children with the highest academic standing. But ten times that number will graduate. What happens to the remainder? What happens to all of those children who scrape through primary school, but would flourish at secondary? There's something truly invidious about five getting a chance at so early an age, while everyone else is deprived.

This issue looms ever larger in the current African experience. It's so serious that it's being discussed at cabinet level in both Zambia and Lesotho. And I well recall a late evening conversation about Uganda that Graça Machel and I had with President Museveni; he was completely stymied by the secondary school dilemma. Graça was making the point, with some considerable animation, that orphan children, in particular, shouldn't be further penalized in life by the denial of secondary education. Museveni didn't disagree. He just didn't know what to do.

As the orphan deluge escalates, education becomes the stuff of life. Africa faces at least two generations of children whose life of the mind, if it was given breath at all, will cease abruptly just as they enter their teens. It's unthinkable. Lost to the world will be hundreds of thousands of creative, gifted, often brilliant spirits. It's happened before in history. Between 1933 and 1945, we lost similar numbers who, had they lived, would have made enormous contributions in every profession, in literature and the arts, in academe, in science, in the entire kaleidoscope of human activity. The holocaust fractured a large piece of civilization. This is a different, but analogous, holocaust.

IV

WOMEN: HALF THE WORLD, BARELY REPRESENTED

ON THE WALL of my study at home, there hangs a picture which I value highly, albeit in a somewhat perverse fashion. It's a stunning photograph of the entire leadership of the United Nations secretariat in 1985. The Secretary-General of the time was Javier Pérez de Cuéllar, surrounded by all of his Under-Secretaries-General and all of his Assistant Secretaries-General. They're standing in a resplendent, unbroken row on the podium of the General Assembly, immediately beneath the huge and ornate representation of the logo of the United Nations.

There are thirty-two of them in all. Not one woman. Not one. It was 1985, a mere twenty years ago.

That just about says everything there is to say about multilateralism and gender. I was Canada's ambassador to the United Nations at the time, and with the full encouragement of the Canadian Ministry of Foreign Affairs, I pursued a very tough line on discrimination against women within the UN system, as well as worldwide gender discrimination on every front.

It was actually quite comical at times. On several occasions, after a series of sturdy speeches making the point, over and over again, that the denial of opportunities for women in the United Nations was appalling, some of my closest diplomatic colleagues would take me to task, cautioning me that Canada was driving the nail through the wall on this particular issue. They'd inelegantly corner me in a corridor, and say something to the effect of "enough already." I would reply, with pugnacious bravado, that I wasn't prepared to cease and desist until equality was achieved (absurd suggestion though that was).

The Canadian badgering, however, was not without value. In the 1980s, the Secretary-General actually defied the protocol of the Boys' Club and appointed a woman, Mercedes Pulido de Briceño of Venezuela, at the level of Assistant Secretary-General, as Coordinator for the Improvement of the Status of Women in the secretariat, to oversee the rights, treatment, and promotion of female employees. The position lasted but three years, from 1985 to 1988. Little of tangible note was accomplished, but it did lead to a collaboration on women's issues with the then Assistant Secretary-General for Human Resources Management, a fellow named Kofi Annan. I think it fair to say that he was the only male member of the secretariat with whom I worked who cared one whit about access and opportunities for women within the United Nations.

It was just prior to Kofi Annan's ascension to the human resources post that Pérez de Cuéllar summoned me to his quarters to say that he had decided to ask Canada to fill a vacant Under-Secretary-General's position in the Department of Public Information, and he and his staff were making the offer to Canada specifically because they were confident we'd appoint a woman.

We did. (Although therein lies a tale. When I exultantly phoned the Ministry of Foreign Affairs to say that Canada would be leading this breakthrough on gender, and to ask whom we might appoint, they had not a single candidate in reserve. It was surreal in a way: here we were, advancing the cause of female appointments within the secretariat, and given the opportunity, we couldn't come up with a name! It was a perfect commentary on the indelible pattern of male privilege: even within the Canadian public service, there were so few women in the upper echelons that when it came to a preferred international appointment, the cupboard was bare.)

What was nuts, of course, is that there were numbers upon numbers of talented women to do the job, but they were invisible, living in the refracted shadows of the glass ceiling. Thus it was that we had a frantic search for a credible appointment. I, myself, made a number of "high-level" calls, but everyone I approached had job commitments they were unable to break or didn't want to break. Finally, a suitable candidate was found: the Canadian government put forward the name of Thérèse Paquet-Sévigny, a vice-president of communications for the CBC. It was, of course, accepted. (Back then, such nominations were always uncritically accepted, and it hasn't changed that much to this day).

The year was 1987. Believe it or not, it was the first permanent appointment of a woman to the post of Under-Secretary-General in the history of the United Nations. Thérèse Paquet-Sévigny's performance was sublimely unmemorable (to my mind perfectly understandable; you need practically a lifetime to master communications within the UN). But that hardly mattered; the barrier had finally been broken.

I want to dwell on this for a bit because it will help to explain why the broader Millennium Development Goal of gender equality has no chance of being reached by 2015.

Fundamentally, the United Nations should be driving the gender agenda. It's the world body with the greatest reach, and everything that underpins its legitimacy speaks to equality. The Charter of the United Nations, the Universal Declaration of Human Rights, the Convention on the Elimination of All Forms of Discrimination Against Women, the Covenant on Economic, Social and Cultural Rights, the Covenant on Political and Civil Rights — they all speak to equality.

Every one of these landmark human rights instruments contains explicit clauses affirming non-discrimination on the basis of sex and declaring equality between men and women. If they were followed, this would be a different world.

Undoubtedly, the covenant with the greatest potential influence is the Convention on the Elimination of All Forms of Discrimination Against Women (CEDAW), which was promulgated on December 18, 1979. It's as though it were the Magna Carta for women. No other convention is quite so powerfully worded. Not only does it aggressively assert equality, but it does so, article by article, in every domain: health, education, justice, social welfare, ad infinitum. It's also the second most highly ratified convention in the history of international covenants: 181 out of 191 countries have ratified. Only the Convention on the Rights of the Child has a larger number of ratifications, at 189. It should also be remembered that when a country ratifies a convention, it effectively becomes an instrument of binding international law in that country. It speaks volumes that so many countries feel they can ignore the prescriptions of CEDAW with impunity; there are simply no enforcement mechanisms, and when it's inconvenient to uphold the convention, countries are blithely negligent.

Let me remind you of Article 3 of the Convention: "States Parties shall take in all fields, in particular in the social, economic and cultural fields, all appropriate measures, including legislation, to ensure the full development and advancement for women, for the purpose of guaranteeing them the exercise and enjoyment of human rights and fundamental freedoms on a basis of equality with men."

What could be more categorical?

In addition to the exemplary covenants of equality, it's also useful to invoke the substance of the great international conferences which were held throughout the 1990s, and actually form the basis for the agenda of the United Nations in the twenty-first century, including the MDGs. It is sometimes forgotten that the world gathered in a successive series of conferences that laboriously etched the mandate for social progress for decades to come.

For the purposes of this discussion, the four most important gatherings were the World Conference on Human Rights in Vienna in 1993; the International Conference on Population and Development in Cairo in 1994; the World Summit for Social Development in Copenhagen in 1995, and the Fourth World Conference on Women in Beijing in 1995.

These were not vast conclaves of disputation and negotiation with little relevance to the real world. These were international conferences which gave rise to cadres of women activists, in one country after another, who then spent the better part of their lives advocating for equality. The global became local with a vengeance. What is not often realized is the way in which these conferences became hotbeds of consciousness-raising for women from all over the developing world, significant numbers of them sponsored to attend by aid agencies and major NGOs. Over those years, our own CIDA paid for hundreds, possibly thousands, of local women activists to attend international gatherings, then return to their home countries to take up the cause. That process continues to this day: at all of the biennial AIDS conferences, for example (the last three were in Durban in 2000, Barcelona in 2002, and Bangkok in 2004, with Toronto scheduled to be the host in August 2006), thousands of women delegates came under the auspices of enlightened sponsors from western countries. The experience is transforming. Everyone returns home determined to light the fires of change. The paucity of progress following those global meetings has had little to do with the women; it has everything to do with the monolithic walls of male authority, and how indescribably tough it is to bring those walls down.

Selected extracts from the conference documents are germane.

From Human Rights in Vienna; the Declaration and Programme of Action:

> Recalling the preamble to the Charter of the United Nations, in particular the determination to reaffirm faith in fundamental human rights, in the dignity and worth of the human person, and in the equal rights of men and women . . .

> [Paragraph 18:] The human rights of women and of the girl-child are an inalienable, integral and indivisible part of universal human rights. The full and equal participation of women in political, civil, economic, social and cultural life . . . and the eradication of all forms of discrimination on grounds of sex are priority objectives of the international community . . .

Having used these quotations, I can't resist saying a word about the Vienna conference itself. I was fortunate enough to attend (with my older daughter), and unlike most such conferences, where the meetings and activities and sessions are a jumble of good-natured chaos, this conclave had one all-consuming, overriding theme that became its mantra: Women's Rights are Human Rights. It was emblazoned on posters in every conference room and corridor, the poster itself depicting women trapped behind a barbed-wire fence of oppression.

The conference activities were actually quite amazing. The women's movement was ferociously well-organized, and determined to shape the debate. The women caucused constantly, and confronted the male-dominated delegations in one spirited exchange after another — not, of course, in the formal conference proceedings (they were reserved for governments), but in separate meetings with the individual delegations, one on one. Gradually, the entire conference shifted agenda: the mantra took hold; the men ran for cover. From namby-pamby declarations of good intent, there emerged a strongly worded document mirroring the best that the international conventions had to offer.

And the conference did something else which was utterly novel and truly memorable. Under the inspired direction of Charlotte Bunch, head of the Center for Women's Global Leadership at Rutgers University, the women activists took one entire day, created a human rights tribunal, and received a horrifying litany of personal testimonies, from thirty-three women representing twenty-five countries, about the physical and sexual violence to which they had been subjected. The massive audience of over a thousand was transformed into a torrent of rage and tears, and the conference was on notice, from that moment forward, never again to be dismissive where the human rights of women were concerned.

But then the conference adjourned, and as is so often the case, all the promises made in the heat of anxiety and fear subsided. The promises were not entirely extinguished; the truth about the women's movement is that it builds, incrementally, from event to event, issue to issue. But it's always a struggle to maintain the momentum.

Let me turn to the Conference on Population and Development in Cairo, and quote from Chapter IV of the Programme of Action, "Gender Equality, Equity and Empowerment of Women":

> The objectives are:
> (a) To achieve equality and equity based on harmonious partnership between men and women and enable women to realize their full potential;
> (b) To ensure the enhancement of women's contributions to sustainable development through their full involvement in policy and decision-making processes at all stages . . . as active decision makers, participants and beneficiaries.

Cairo was an epic conference in many respects. Again I was fortunate to be there and to watch the interplay of forces. The conference was chaired by Dr. Nafis Sadik, who was then the executive director of the United Nations Population Fund (UNFPA), and is now, coincidentally, the UN special envoy on HIV/AIDS in Asia. She was superb as she adroitly steered the conference in two significant directions. First, she frontally and courageously locked horns with the Vatican, preventing it from writing an anti-abortion plank into the platform. Second, she subsumed the old definition of family planning into a vastly broader compendium of women's rights, essentially arguing that women's empowerment on all fronts would do as much and more for stabilizing population as any traditional forms of family planning. It's not that contraception was diminished; it was expanded significantly.

But it was not Nafis alone. The conference participants were time and again electrified by the magnificent feminist Bella Abzug, ever-commanding and persuasive. Whenever Bella ventured forth into the corridors, or into the halls where the sessions were held (often sitting in a wheelchair because she was recovering from treatment for cancer, a wheelchair I sometimes joyously pushed), the scene was positively hilarious. It was like some triumphant passage of a reigning matriarch. And as she proceeded through the crowds, words leaping madly in every direction, whole delegations parted like the sea, bowing and scraping and fawning reverentially. What Bella decreed, the conference embraced. Between them, Nafis Sadik and Bella Abzug drove the conference and dictated the outcome.

Next, a quote from the document that emerged from the conference on social development in Copenhagen:

> [A. Paragraph 7:] We acknowledge that social and economic development cannot be secured in a sustainable way without the full participation of women, and that equality and equity between women and men is a priority

for the international community and as such must be at the centre of economic and social development.

And finally, from the Beijing Mission Statement:

[Paragraph 1:] The Platform for Action is an agenda for women's empowerment. It aims at . . . removing all the obstacles to women's active participation in all spheres of public and private life through a full and equal share in economic, social, cultural and political decision-making. This means that the principle of shared power and responsibility should be established between men and women at home, in the workplace and in the wider national and international communities. Equality between women and men is a matter of human rights and a condition for social justice and is also a necessary and fundamental prerequisite for equality, development and peace.

Beijing, of course, was the ne plus ultra for the women's movement. No other conclave in recent memory delivered such a powerful testament of human rights for women. But the experience of Beijing was also desperately difficult for the leadership of the women's movement. Allow me to explain.

The government of China was positively paranoid about the sudden onslaught of thousands of women activists. They wanted the conference, but they wanted it as a showcase and a boon to the economy, not as a hotbed of militant (and I use "militant" in the best sense) advocacy. One of the features of all the previous conferences had been the growing place of grassroots activists. Every international conference, starting with the conference on the environment in Rio in 1992, had had an active NGO component. In every instance, a physical place, called the NGO Forum, and a great deal of time were set aside for the involvement of hordes of participants representing "civil society," the name now given to the full constellation of non-governmental and private voluntary organizations, community groups, charities, advocates and activists, faith-based organizations, and sometimes the private sector.

Twenty-five to thirty thousand women representing civil society were expected in Beijing. The government, recoiling with neurotic palpitations, decided to place the NGO Forum in a suburb called Huairou, some fifty-five kilometres from the actual site of the conference. It was preposterous. The women's movement was up in arms, but to absolutely no avail. There was not a single member government of the United Nations that was prepared to take up the cudgels on their behalf. Does that not speak volumes? It is ever thus: The women's movement rallies, but can find few or no allies amongst the male political establishment, especially if the subject matter is controversial.

I remember it well because I was personally involved in endless strategy meetings (all of them futile) to attempt to reverse the decision of the Chinese government. In advance of Beijing, I had been appointed by the then Secretary-General, Boutros Boutros-Ghali, to the UN Secretary-General's Advisory Group on the Fourth World Conference on Women in Beijing. There were ten of us on the advisory group, and we met in the most wildly improbable of places including (courtesy of Princess Basma Bint Talal of Jordan, who was a member of the group), Petra, Jordan, that absolutely amazing archaeological wonder of the world. We flew into Petra on military helicopters in formation (I was terrified), and presumably the splendid isolation of the place was to endow us with that strategic prescience necessary to bring the government of China to its senses. No such luck. We failed, just as the few others who bothered to try failed.

It is an incomparable tribute to the women's movement that despite the tortured manipulations of China's government, they still managed, even from a distance, to influence the workings of the conference to the extent that a remarkably cogent document emerged. The quote above merely gives the flavour.

Nonetheless, despite these sterling and repeated exhortations for equality, we haven't, in the aftermath, begun to overcome the discrimination, the indignity, the violence visited upon women around the world on a daily basis. Why? Because once consensus is reached and the activists disperse, no major international body steps up to maintain the cohesion and sustain the momentum. Where the rights and needs of women are concerned, the gap between rhetoric and reality remains a yawning chasm. Earlier on, I had expressed the view that the United Nations should be driving the gender agenda. On a daily basis, the UN should be identifying, investigating, documenting, and accusing those who are involved — especially governments — in the continuing systemic discrimination against women. It doesn't happen for a wide variety of reasons.

Despite all the lip service paid by the UN member states to the importance of gender equality, only 11 of the 191 ambassadors, or 5.7 percent, are women. Worse still, the make-up of the workforce of the UN agencies — a balance over which the powers-that-be within the secretariat have some control — is similarly distorted. The funds, programs, and agencies will tell you, proudly, that up to 33 percent of their professional staff are women, but quite aside from asking why it should be only 33 percent (it's both embarrassing and indefensible, the way in which we've consigned 50 percent to some unattainable fantasy), a closer scrutiny will show that the concentration of women is invariably at the lower professional grades. There is enormous talent in these junior professional categories, but inevitably, in the absence of rigorous affirmative action, their movement upwards is halting and incremental. What is more, at this moment of writing, men head the UN Development Programme, the World Health Organization, UNESCO, the World Food Programme, the UN's Food and Agriculture Organization (FAO), the High Commission for Refugees, the International Labour Organization (ILO), the UN Office on Drugs and Crime, the World Bank, the International Monetary Fund, UNAIDS and the United Nations Environment Programme. Women head UNICEF, the UNFPA, the High Commission for Human Rights, and UN-Habitat. There are, to be sure, lesser and smaller agencies, but these are the important ones. The imbalance is striking — and representative.

But that's just the half of it, and the lesser half. The other aspect of multilateralism, astonishing and offensive in equal measure, is the absence of any single, powerful agency within the UN system to represent women. Women constitute more than half the world's population, and in the extensive labyrinth of UN organizations, they are barely represented.

I say "barely" because there is the United Nations Development Fund for Women, or UNIFEM, as it's known. Its headquarters in New York has a core staff of between forty-five and fifty, with a number of non-permanent staff and consultants posted here and there internationally (a ludicrously small number on the entire African continent). UNICEF, representing the children of the world, has 8,311 full-time staff, a cornucopia of consultants and ample offices in over 150 countries. Please understand: UNIFEM is supposed to represent the women of the world with an annual core budget that was $45 million in 2004. UNICEF had an annual budget that hovered close to $2 billion in 2004. (That's a ratio of over 40 to 1.)

The UNFPA does address women in significant ways, but mostly on targeted issues of family planning and sexual and reproductive health. Its mandate is far too narrow to pretend to deal with the vast array of women's concerns, and rather like UNIFEM, it is wildly underfunded for the job it wants to do. Partly because it's been financially penalized by the Bush administration — on grounds that UNFPA was promoting abortion in China, grounds so dishonest as to be actionable — UNFPA has barely a fifth of the finances of UNICEF.

All the other agencies named above tend to deal with themes — governance, health, education, food, housing, and so on — and do not dwell, with any consuming focus, on women.

No, if women were to be taken seriously, it would be via UNIFEM. But UNIFEM is little known beyond UN circles, and is not taken seriously by the hierarchy within. How could it be? Apart from the minuscule budget, neither the executive director of UNIFEM, nor UNIFEM itself, is senior on the UN grid; it's so embarrassing and so objectionable that I can barely talk about it with equanimity.

UNIFEM is not a free-standing agency. It's simply a section or division of the UNDP, and the woman who heads it is eclipsed in status by many of her UNDP colleagues working in other divisions. In fact, she's superceded in standing not only by every single other agency head in the UN family, but by every special representative (my part-time self included) appointed by the Secretary-General. In a system where hierarchy is everything, where everyone defers to the person above in the twisted gradations of bureaucratic aristocracy, to be at the level of the head of UNIFEM — a D2, it's called — is to have no greater status than, say, a person who heads up a UNICEF office in one large country.

But this isn't a large country we're talking about. We're talking about more than half the world's population. And it's rank, really rank, to treat women's issues in such a scandalous manner. Let me make it clear: In my over twenty years working directly or indirectly with the United Nations, I can safely say that only a tiny cadre of voices speaks strongly for women. Admittedly, it has proven next to impossible to get the member countries to work towards the advancement of women; they always have such mixed and freighted motivation. But nothing excuses the dilatory indifference of the UN agency leadership.

I'm speaking this strongly because the matter has been closeted for long enough, my views on it are well-known, and they are views for which I will never apologize. It seems to me absolutely inexcusable that women have been given such short shrift in the UN constellation. And please spare me the defensive assertions that the agencies themselves look after women's issues, that the issues are "mainstreamed" into the agendas of the agencies. First of all, I've travelled more than most people from country to country, and I'm prepared to argue till doomsday with anyone who pretends that women are a top priority in UN agencies' country programming. They never have been and are not to this day. The proof is in the reality: just look at the toll that AIDS has taken on women.

Instead of bona fide, specialized programs, women get "gender mainstreaming," and gender mainstreaming is a pox for women. The worst thing you can do for women is to fold their concerns into the mandates of UN agencies, or bury them under the activities of government ministries. Once you've mainstreamed gender, it's everybody's business and nobody's business. Everyone's accountable and no one's accountable. I don't know who thought up this mainstreaming guff, but I often wonder what the motives were. And even if the motives were well-meaning, surely experience has proved how damaging to women mainstreaming truly is. We've mainstreamed women's needs into some kind of shibboleth, and can someone tell me how those needs have been better served by doing so?

Gender mainstreaming might work if we had what the sports and financial enthusiasts call a "level playing field," that is to say, if there were real equity and equality between women and men. Then gender mainstreaming becomes a way of maintaining that equality. But when you start from such gross inequality, mainstreaming simply entrenches the disparities. Hence the need for a totally separate vehicle to carry women's rights forward until that hallowed day (I can practically hear the chorus of hallelujahs rising up behind me) when equality is achieved.

So the only way to deal with these issues is to preserve for them pride of place — to construct for women an edifice, an institution, an agency whose sole preoccupation is to advance the position of women. Or more accurately, to support women to create their own such entity. Then you couldn't mainstream, mute, or dilute it in any way because it would be separate — separately responsible, separately accountable. Its voice would always be heard because it wouldn't be subsumed into the miasma of uniformity.

Ah, yes, some will say, but you're missing something, Mr. Lewis. Isn't there a Division for the Advancement of Women (DAW) right in the secretariat, cheek by jowl with the Office of the Secretary-General? The answer is yes, although, like many others, I've never been sure what the office actually does. Presumably it is a liaison point with treaty bodies and commissions, serving as the secretariat for some conferences, and advising the Secretary-General when advice is felt to be needed.

The senior position in DAW is registered at the level of Assistant Secretary-General, a significant notch above that of the executive director of UNIFEM. I can say with confidence that when I last stopped paying attention, instead of a productive and energetic collaboration between the offices, there was nothing but bad blood. At its most absurdly elemental, DAW didn't want any prominence for UNIFEM, and played interference wherever possible. And UNIFEM, understandably, devoted a great deal of time and energy fighting back. It was nuts, really, because UNIFEM was operational and DAW was conceptual; there should never have been any competition, except that destructive internal rivalries are the nemesis of UN functioning.

Now let me say, before proceeding further, that I must record what some would deem a conflict of interest: my daughter, a human rights lawyer, worked for UNIFEM for seven years before returning to Canada. But frankly, you will simply have to accept that I'm capable of making measured judgements regardless the delicious frippery of coincidental connection.

I readily acknowledge that a lot of what I've described as evidence of cosmic indifference to women is internal United Nations and process stuff. But process is important because it prejudices everything else. For example, take a look at the MDGS themselves. The third goal, the one that deals with gender, measures the attainment of equality by establishing a target to "Eliminate gender disparity in primary and secondary education, preferably by 2005, and in all levels of education no later than 2015." Now, how curious is that? Were there no other indices available? Since when did equality and empowerment of women rest solely on gender disparity *in primary and secondary school*? It's frankly ridiculous. What happened to the measures of equality as defined in all the conventions, in terms of every aspect of civil, economic, social, and political life?

To be sure, when it came to publishing the Millennium Task Force monograph on that particular goal (every goal had a task force), the measures were expanded to include all the usual suspects, from property rights to sexual violence. But why was all of that not part of the original goals and targets, since the prescription for achieving gender equality had been set out unequivocally in both the Cairo and Beijing Programmes of Action? The drafters of the MDGS were a thousand times better on the myriad targets for the goal on the environment, and the goal on global partnerships, than they were for the goal on women. I'm writing this in advance of the debate on the MDGS at the United Nations in September 2005, but there is not a scintilla of doubt in my mind that the needs and rights of women will receive short shrift. Nothing in the preparation for the debate leads me to believe that anything has changed. The world's governments will make the required comments, and then pretend that words alone stop violence, end oppression, and guarantee economic opportunity. There is no greater emblem of international hypocrisy than the promise of women's rights.

And there is no more reprehensible "oversight" than what was missing completely from the mix of MDGS from the outset — namely, a goal for sexual and reproductive rights. It wasn't explicitly identified under gender equality or touched upon under maternal mortality, and yet it constitutes one of the great issues of our time. Again I ask, how could that happen? Easy: When so few in the secretariat or in the agencies have the power (or inclination) to influence policy around women, the issues are easily slighted.

I well remember a meeting in June 2004, under the auspices of the Rockefeller Foundation, held at their headquarters, designed to somehow overcome this glaring omission within the MDGS. Peter Piot, the executive director of UNAIDS was there, as was Thoraya Obaid, the executive director of UNFPA. So, too, everyone from the head of the population council to the minister of health of Namibia. The focus of the meeting was to figure out why the communities dealing with HIV/AIDS on the one hand, and the communities dealing with sexual and reproductive health on the other, functioned in such discrete silos when tackling sexually transmitted diseases. It made no sense. They should be working in integrated harmony.

That case was most eloquently made by Thoraya Obaid, clearly smarting from the marginalization of the issues that form the mandate for her agency. In a carefully worded statement, Thoraya made the case for the integration of HIV/AIDS and sexual and reproductive health, noting, with regret, that the two operated in separate compartments, which made no sense whatsoever. Both, after all, required dealing in significant ways with all the difficult issues raised by sexually transmitted diseases. Much of the subsequent discussion bemoaned the absence of sexual and reproductive health from the MDGS, and several participants argued that the HIV/AIDS MDG provided the vehicle through which sexual and reproductive health could be thrust into the vortex of the MDG debate.

It was evident that everyone hoped that the meeting would stimulate a far more widespread discussion of sexual and reproductive health, whenever and wherever the MDGS were being addressed. It didn't really matter whether that happened within the context of AIDS, or poverty, or maternal mortality, so long as it happened. I don't doubt, therefore, that sexual and reproductive health will occupy a significant place at the UN Millennium debate in September 2005. But it's absurd — if symptomatic — to have to insert an issue of such centrality into the mix in so roundabout a fashion.

It reminds me of the unsuccessful attempts made by UNIFEM to become one of the co-sponsoring agencies of UNAIDS. There are ten co-sponsors, everyone from UNESCO and UNICEF to WFP and the ILO. Unfortunately, however, there was no room for UNIFEM: the women of the world had to settle for a memorandum of understanding with the UNAIDS secretariat. Undoubtedly it was argued that

UNIFEM, as a division of UNDP, was already represented. Forgive me, but it says something about the way the rights of women are viewed within the UN family that a procedural, but entirely contrived argument should prevail.

There's just no way around the constant neglect in addressing the priorities for women. Perhaps the most recent glaring example of that truth is the report of the celebrated Commission for Africa, appointed by Prime Minister Tony Blair.

I can't get over it. Let's start with the commissioners. There were seventeen in total, three of whom were women. Three, or 17 percent. Prime Minister Blair had the whole world to choose from, and he could come up with only three women. Tony Blair claims to be a social democrat; socialists are supposed to have greater sensitivity to such matters. But you see, when it comes to women, sensitivity goes out the window. That commission was fatally flawed from the outset, simply by way of gender representation.

And the report showed it. This is a report that ploughed new ground on foreign aid, on debt, on trade, on climate. It was justly saluted on all those issues for the sweep of its progressive recommendations in areas where others had always feared to tread. It recommended an immediate doubling of foreign aid, a cancellation of the debts of the poorest countries, and a vast reduction in agricultural subsidies as the centrepiece of a new trading regimen. Everyone applauded. As a matter of fact, the report even went so far as to challenge the intellectual underpinnings of the World Bank and the International

Monetary Fund in their dual adherence to fundamentalist monetarism. On all those fronts it was bold, oh so bold.

But on women? The report is an absolute throwback. Other than the occasional paragraphs paying obligatory obeisance to women's rights, there's a feckless failure to recognize that women sustain the entire continent of Africa, and should have a definitive role in every single aspect of social, economic, political, civil, and cultural life, from peacekeeping to agriculture to trade to AIDS. If there had been a Commission for Africa with fourteen women and three men, I can absolutely guarantee that the final report would have differed root and branch from the report we now have in hand. One day — probably in the next millennium — such a commission will be appointed.

And just to demonstrate the absolute, unwavering consistency in such matters, allow me to mention, however heretical it may seem, the communiqué issued in July 2005 by the G8 meeting in Gleneagles. Honestly, it's like a parody. From my impeccable desktop printer, the document emerges as eighteen pages in length, thirty-five paragraphs in all, five thousand to six thousand words, with two full appendices. There are five references to women: two in that most common linguistic fusion of "women and children," one mandatory reference to "pregnant women and babies," one in conjunction with youth employment, and one throwaway line, entirely neutral, incorporating "gender equality." It is my contention — a contention with which many commentators would take issue — that the stunning absence of emphasis on women in the official pronouncement of the G8 is an ominous omen for the delivery of commitments made. You simply cannot be serious about Africa and treat women with such contempt. It won't work. Mark my words: Come 2010, G8 excuses will be the order of the day. Bush, Blair, Chirac, Schroeder, perhaps even Martin, will all be out to pasture, shrugging shoulders of insouciance. Read the document, note the void, and weep.

But when all is said and done, the ongoing struggle to embrace gender equality was most poignantly brought home to me in confronting the pandemic of HIV/AIDS. And in particular, one specific memorable experience.

In January 2003, I travelled with James Morris, the executive director of the World Food Programme, to four countries in southern Africa: Zimbabwe, Malawi, Zambia, and Lesotho. Southern Africa was then (as now) in the grip of a brutal food shortage, and the combination of hunger and AIDS was something we wanted to investigate. Apart from the evidence of catastrophe which was flowing from the reports of UN representatives in the field, there was also a newly current academic thesis called "New Variant Famine." The name had been coined by Alex de Waal, a gifted and knowledgeable Africanist, who, upon close study, had evolved the argument that food shortages were the result of illness caused by AIDS as much as they were the result of climate.

We were interested, if skeptical. It seemed far more likely that the driving force would be erratic rainfall and drought.

I had been in the region only the month before, and experienced a kind of renewable shock, but James Morris, on his first extensive trip to the region, was absolutely stunned by what we encountered. There was hunger and starvation everywhere, and while the actual famine or near-famine was clearly influenced by successive droughts, there was no question that AIDS was playing havoc with agricultural productivity. So many farmers — overwhelmingly women — were sick, or had died, or were busy coping with the dying and orphaned, that they simply couldn't have tilled the fields, tended to the crops, or gone to market, even had the weather patterns been hospitable.

The state of the health of the women in the villages was ghastly. Household income was ransacked, and time once spent on walking to distant fields and growing a variety of foods had been given over to caring for the sick. AIDS leads to hunger; hunger exacerbates AIDS. It's a merciless interaction. The numbers of orphan children are beyond belief, in fact, so beyond belief that when we drafted our report, we actually said, "The situation of orphans represents a humanitarian catastrophe and a violation of the rights of children. The apparent inability of the United Nations system and the international community to adequately support national governments in their response to the needs of the huge numbers of orphans in the region is unacceptable." That's UN-speak for saying, "You've failed lamentably: for God's sake get your act together."

We travelled with eighteen colleagues from eight different UN agencies and the Southern African Development Community (SADC), and I vividly remember the repetitive sense of numbed incomprehension as we boarded the WFP plane to fly to yet another country.

One of those travelling colleagues was my advisor on women's issues, Paula Donovan. Paula and I had worked together at UNICEF headquarters for four years, and after I left, she'd headed off to Nairobi as regional advisor for UNICEF's AIDS programming in East and southern Africa. Having her on the trip with Jim Morris meant that the situation of women was always front and centre, and it was Paula who ultimately drafted the sections on women of the final report which were so tough and so trenchant. If she had not been along, our indignation and concern would undoubtedly have been expressed in more muted terms. Considering what flowed from the report, it was a piece of extraordinary good fortune that her pen and her conscience were at hand.

Let me quote the key paragraph at some little length:

> The mission was struck in particular by how food shortages appear to aggravate the impact of HIV/AIDS by accelerating the progress of the disease in HIV-positive individuals . . . Perhaps the most disturbing realization came with a better understanding of the impact that this crisis is having on the region's women. It was evident to the mission that although the prevalence of HIV infection is highest among women and girls — who also take on nearly all the responsibilities of caring for the sick and orphaned, in addition to their regular obligations such as providing food for their households — very little is being done to reduce women's

> risks, to protect them from sexual aggression and violence, to ease their burdens or to support their coping and caring efforts. The apparent lack of urgency, leadership, direction and responsibility in the response of the United Nations, national governments, and the international community to the pandemic's effects on women and girls is deeply troubling. For example, the early adoption of mainstreaming approaches to gender within United Nations agencies, funds and programmes has made gender issues everyone's concern but no one's responsibility. Whereas gender policies and principles are widely discussed by the United Nations, governments and NGOs, the urgent actions flowing from those discussions must be implemented. So far, that does not appear to have happened.

When we drafted our final press release, we abandoned the measured language and made the findings even louder and more conclusive: "While responding to the severe food crisis in southern Africa, an even greater disaster has been unearthed. The HIV/AIDS pandemic is compounding the premature death of thousands of productive people — particularly women — across the region, and is wrecking the livelihoods of millions more while sowing the seeds of future famines . . . The incredible assault of HIV/AIDS on women in particular has no parallel in human history. Women are the pillars of the family and community — the mothers, the care-givers, the farmers. The pandemic is preying on them relentlessly, threatening them in a way that the world has never yet witnessed."

So shaken were we by what we'd seen that upon our return we appealed to the Secretary-General to intervene. On my part, it wasn't the first time. He would be more than ready to acknowledge, I believe, that I had raised the plight of women over and over again in the preceding year and a half. In fact, yet again it leads me to a digression which, in this instance, I cannot resist.

Earlier on, at the end of October of 2002, on one of my regular reporting visits to the Secretary-General, I had raised the question of the excruciating vulnerability of women in the face of AIDS. In July of that year, at the international AIDS conference in Barcelona, I had observed during a press conference that "the toll on women and girls is beyond imagining; it presents Africa and the world with a practical and moral challenge which places gender at the centre of the human condition . . . For the African continent, it means economic and social survival. For the women and girls of Africa, it's a matter of life and death." I was consumed by what was happening to women (and there are virtually no improvements to this day; if anything, things are worse); anyone would have been similarly consumed. Everywhere I went it was a scene out of Dante.

On this particular occasion in the fall of 2002, my plea to the Secretary-General was this: I told him that with his permission, I was prepared to draft a plan of action for the United Nations to respond to the predicament of women. I argued that further amassing of evidence was unnecessary; what was desperately needed was intervention. He agreed. In fact, he went further. I remember it well because he said that I should proceed, but make sure that the plan was long-term, and that he himself felt so strongly about the issue that he would go out and raise money to make sure that the plan could be implemented. (He even mentioned the Gates Foundation as a possible source.)

I left feeling quite elated, determined to put something on paper as quickly as possible. I was more than somewhat surprised, therefore, when, a week or ten days later, I got a call from the office of the Deputy Secretary-General inviting me to join a meeting (given my schedule, I joined by conference call) to discuss, amongst other things, the response to women and AIDS in Africa. There were a number of people on the call (it was eventually held on November 22), including Mark Malloch Brown, then head of UNDP, Eveline Herfkens, the Secretary-General's coordinator of the MDG campaign working through UNDP, Peter Piot, head of UNAIDS, one or two aides from the thirty-eighth floor (as the offices of the Secretary-General were known), and me. The meeting was chaired by Louise Fréchette, the Deputy Secretary-General.

The conversation meandered from women, to the role of civil society, to the general raising of money for UN priorities (I was quite baffled about the content, although I participated when asked), and at the close, Louise Fréchette assigned — I repeat, assigned — Eveline Herfkens and Peter Piot the job of jointly coming up with a plan to address the question of women and AIDS. I did not protest. It was not my place to protest. It was clear that the understanding I'd struck with the Secretary-General had been superceded by the specific assignment of the Deputy Secretary-General.

This actually raises a point with which I've often wrestled. To what extent should I put up a fight with the powers-that-be? It's a very tough call. I've always felt that the work I do is taken seriously by the United Nations, but never quite seriously enough to override the normal bureaucratic rhythms. I knew that I had been finessed on the women's issue, but I felt that I could still influence it from other points on the UN compass and beyond, rather than causing a ruckus internally, getting nowhere, and alienating everyone along the way.

To be fair, it may well be that upon further reflection on the thirty-eighth floor, it was felt that I was not the appropriate person to draw up a draft proposal for any kind of planned response. After all, I had no institutional base: I was a part-time envoy, reporting to the Secretary-General, but working very much on my own. It may also have been felt that I was too radical in my views and pronouncements. Whatever the assumption, I was effectively taken out of the mix.

What deeply troubled me at the time, however, was my conviction that nothing would come of the alternative. Success would require the engagement of all the major agencies, not to speak of governments and other partners. Eveline was relatively new to the UN bureaucracy, and though she had been an inspired minister of international co-operation in the Dutch cabinet in a previous incarnation, she would need time to figure out the

Byzantine ways of the United Nations. Peter Piot was, at that very moment, running for the job of director general of the WHO in a very difficult race, and it was frankly absurd to imagine that he could possibly find the time to help fashion an entirely new approach to an issue of such complexity and importance. In fact, he was on the verge of announcing a leave of absence to focus on his campaign.

In the upshot, I never heard another word of it again. And the fact that nothing came of it was manifest in the need two months later, in early 2003, to raise the issue all over again. I would argue that this is what always happens where the rights and needs of women are concerned: an inexplicable willingness to let things slide, an inescapable drift to inertia.

But James Morris and I couldn't allow institutional rigor mortis to set in after what we had just seen in southern Africa — not after our joint horror at the plight of women — and so we appealed to Secretary-General Annan to take unprecedented action.

And he did. He called a meeting in February, which was held in the small conference room adjacent to his office. He assembled a number of heads of agencies and his own senior people headed by Iqbal Riza, his chief of staff. He also had James Morris on teleconference from Rome, with other UN dignitaries from Geneva. I was asked to comment and did so as feelingly as I could summon. But the main intervention came from James Morris who, because of his standing as head of a major agency, made a tremendous impact on everyone. With quiet eloquence, he drew a picture of women and orphans so beset by pain and trauma that the United Nations must surely intervene. The tide was turned, or so it seemed.

The Secretary-General, fully seized of the imperative, said that he wanted to strike a task force and looked anxiously around the table for someone to chair it. Catherine Bertini, James Morris's predecessor at the WFP, and the then Under-Secretary-General for Management, said that no doubt Carol Bellamy, the executive director of UNICEF, would want to chair it and should be appointed. Carol Bellamy was not there, but the Secretary-General agreed, and on the spot struck the task force with Bellamy in charge.

It took an inordinate amount of time to get things going, but eventually it was decided to promulgate the Secretary-General's Task Force on Women, Girls and HIV/AIDS in Southern Africa, and to begin by studying the situation in nine countries. Originally, of course, it was meant to be a worldwide plan of action, or one focused at least on the whole continent of Africa. But somehow, it all got whittled down. (It's odd, though: everything the United Nations undertakes expands in Topsyesque fashion — everything, that is, except initiatives on women.)

Over several months in 2004, the study proceeded with the participation of many excellent people in the countries concerned, and the report was released in July 2004. It's actually a very good document, and if anything comes of it, real strides might be made. But as of this writing, very little has come of it, and the situation for women remains as perilous as ever.

On a number of occasions, in subsequent visits to several of the nine countries covered by the report, I've raised the question of whether or not the recommendations have been or will be implemented. In some countries, there's even a program of action following on the report, but as yet there's no funding available. And just as a wearying footnote, the United Nations also lost Sisonke Msimang, a truly remarkable young African woman, responsible for large parts of the task force report, who was based at the United Nations in Johannesburg, and who might have single-handedly made implementation possible if she'd had the necessary support from within the UN system. It didn't come. In a spirit of considerable regret, she left to work for George Soros, but it's a huge loss. And it's a further commentary on the multilateral priorities for women.

I never feel more agitated than in the face of what's happening to women. The atmosphere of benign neglect, compounded by the rooted gender inequality, all adds up to a death sentence for countless millions of women in the developing world. For whatever reason, we can't break the monolith of indifference and paralysis.

I've tried in this lecture to give you a glimpse, experienced or discerned on a personal basis, of the struggle for women's human rights. I can't pretend that it's more than a glimpse, and it doesn't begin to approximate the frustrations and heroism, tenacity and despair, progress and setbacks faced by the leaders of the women's movement itself. I've concentrated on Africa, as I have before in these lectures, because it's the continent I know best, and because it yields such vivid examples.

Governments in Africa do not do well in the protection of women's rights. In fact, as I shall momentarily demonstrate, they are profoundly deficient. I've been completely taken aback, on more than one occasion, by the wall of indifference thrown up by cabinet ministers when I raise, for example, the plight of women in the era of AIDS. At one point, in the case of Angola, a very senior member of the administration lapsed into locker-room smirking at the mere mention of women. My argument is quite simple: They would not be allowed to indulge in such asinine and/or negligent behaviour if there were a watchdog, a full-fledged agency or institution as part of the United Nations, whose job it was to ride herd on the recalcitrants. Governments get away with it because no one cares enough to prevent governments from getting away with it.

And what is the upshot? In the UNDP Human Development Report for 2003, there is a gender-related development index which rates most of the countries of the world according to a number of economic and social indices, taking into account, in particular, performance on the overall status of women. Let me identify the 20 countries at the bottom of the list of 145 which are ranked for gender, starting with the country right at the bottom, and working up: Sierra Leone, Niger, Burkina Faso, Mali, Burundi, Mozambique, Ethiopia, Central African Republic, Guinea-Bissau, Democratic Republic of the

Congo, Angola, Côte d'Ivoire, Chad, Zambia, Malawi, Benin, Tanzania, Rwanda, Senegal, Eritrea.

Twenty countries. All are African. While it is appalling that Africa occupies a place of such dishonour, showing how so many leaders are beyond redemption on issues of gender, it should also give everyone pause about the role of multilateralism. It's not possible for the UN family in any of these twenty countries to grab the heads of state by the scruff of the neck and shake them into equality. But it should be the role of the UN family to shame, blame, and propose solutions, all the while yelling from the rooftops that inequality is obscene. Only then will change have a chance.

V

SOLUTIONS: A GALLERY OF ALTERNATIVES IN GOOD FAITH

THE ESSENCE OF these lectures is not difficult to divine: the Millennium Development Goals will not be reached in Africa. As I explored the issues dealt with in the previous four lectures, it became more and more apparent that without dramatic change, the goals are an intellectual illusion. We are in a desperate race against time, and we're losing. It's simply impossible to reduce poverty, hunger, gender inequality, disease, and death significantly at the present pace, and other than the contrapuntal beat of hyperactive rhetoric, the necessary acceleration is nowhere evident.

Alas, man and woman cannot live by rhetoric alone.

That being the case, what I would like to do in this final lecture is to advance a number of ideas, possibilities, suggestions, recommendations, solutions, which, were they to be applied to Africa, in whole or in part, would give the continent a much better chance of survival. Some of the suggestions are sound; some are unselfconsciously eccentric, some will be seen as implausible. In certain instances, I highlight initiatives that are already in place, but which carry high levels of risk or uncertainty, requiring a special declaration of support. I offer them all as a gallery of alternatives in good faith. I would offer almost anything as an antidote to the pathetically blinkered and unimaginative current approach which holds the continent in thrall.

First, then, let me address the G8 Summit. Something occurred at the July 2005 Summit at Gleneagles in Scotland that was deeply regrettable. Because of all the hype, because of the Live 8 spectacle, because of the Madison Avenue role of Geldof (Bono was much more measured), and above all, because of the brilliant co-option of the NGO community by Tony Blair, civil society was effectively muzzled in its response. Its normally tough, analytic appraisals were replaced by adoring complicity; the principled NGO community suddenly found itself basking in the incestuous aura of power. It was as if everyone was in the same tent, while Tony Blair did his laying on of hands. Most of the major NGO players knew that they'd been had, but there was a wilful contagion of laryngitis. To read their press releases was almost comical: the words lay leaden on the page. They could barely summon a twitch of indignation, let alone a spasm of outrage.

It was the first time that I can remember when, for civil society, half a loaf was better than a full loaf. They congratulated the G8 on progress made, overstated that progress, and then uttered only the most plaintive pleas for more.

Let me offer a rather different response. This is what should now happen: The Jubilee Coalition — the international alliance of religious groups and other activists who've done such a superb job driving the cancellation of debt — should, on an emergency basis, be expanded into a coalition on the cancellation of agricultural subsidies. The first target is the World Trade Organization meeting in Hong Kong in December 2005; the lobbying between now and then should be furious. We're in real trouble on trade: the prospects are bleak. Unless there is a break in the impasse at Hong Kong, unless the European Union and the United States do a *volte-face* on agricultural subsidies, this round of the WTO talks is effectively doomed, and with it, Africa's access to international markets.

On debt, the existing coalition should go flat out for the cancellation of all remaining African debt — still over $200 billion — for all countries. The modest progress at Gleneagles —- $40 billion for eighteen countries, fourteen of them African — should be seen as a foot in the door, rather than a major achievement. We have to break the pattern of obsequious rejoicing for every incremental fraction.

On Official Development Assistance, what is needed is a year-by-year accounting of individual G8 contributions. This business of doubling aid by 2010, or tripling aid by 2015, just doesn't work. What happens in the intervening years when there are no interim goals? The world has to be made to understand that the targets set at

Gleneagles are critically flawed on two grounds: they won't be reached and they're not high enough.

Consider this: The G8 countries vowed that they would double annual aid to Africa by 2010, that is, another $25 billion a year. But UNAIDS has recently released a definitive report indicating that by 2008, two years before that deadline, HIV/AIDS alone will require $22 billion a year, most of it for African countries. What immediately becomes clear is that the G8 target is unacceptably low. Where is the money for poverty, hunger, education, water, sanitation, nutrition, malaria, tuberculosis, other diseases, the fight against infant and maternal mortality, and environmental sustainability? They needed an extra $50 billion a year by 2010, not $25 billion, and they were afraid to ask for it. Afraid, even though the $50 billion would simply reflect the target of 0.7 percent of GNP to which all western governments are supposedly committed. The pittance promised by the United States, doubling $3 billion annually (the current U.S. level of aid to Africa) to $6 billion by 2010, instead of the $16 billion which would represent their fair share, dooms the G8 bargain.

It's the old story: Set your sights low enough to increase your chances of success and hope that no one notices.

It really drives me to distraction. We fill the stage with raucous applause because the G8 Summit gives the appearance of delivering large sums of money, and indeed, there is more money. But what no one seems willing to admit is that the abysmal amounts of Official

Development Assistance over the last decade have so prejudiced the integrity of Africa that the larger sums now promised won't begin to compensate for the history of neglect.

The G8 countries talk extravagantly, but Gleneagles ultimately failed to deliver. Had the NGO community not been so fettered by political flim-flam, there would have been a proper international uproar. If this were a serious world, rather than a world of thinly disguised neo-colonial manipulation, the G8 would have moved to fulfill its thirty-six-year-old promise of contributing the full 0.7 percent of each country's GNP annually by 2010.

Gordon Brown, the U.K. minister of finance has said, "When there are thirty thousand children dying every day, and when there are one hundred million children not going to school at all in the poorest countries, the need to act is obvious." He's absolutely right, of course. But what about all the years when the need was equally obvious, and the donor world raised hardly a finger? What about all the years since 1990, when the Convention on the Rights of the Child came into effect as an instrument of binding international law — subsequently ratified by nearly every country in the world — and no one paid attention? I'm not such an oaf as to diminish the achievement of modest additional foreign aid; it's important. But it should be accompanied by expressions of abject, near-grovelling apology, not by expressions of insufferable self-congratulation.

And there's something else that must change about the way in which the world works. At the eleventh hour at Gleneagles, the Japanese government, which had been resisting an increase in its annual contribution, suddenly promised to double aid to Africa in three years. It's actually a relative pittance since, as I noted in the first lecture, Japan gives so little now (approximately $1.5 billion a year), and everyone recognized that Japan's sudden change of heart was tied directly to its pursuit of a seat on the Security Council. I would like to propose, therefore, that when and if Japan is elected to the Security Council, there be a written caveat which says that if the money to Africa is not identifiably doubled by July 31, 2008, Japan forfeits its seat. Undoubtedly, that would unleash the winds of consternation, but it would also serve notice that the betrayal of the commitments made to Africa over the years will no longer be tolerated.

Now inevitably, I've begun this array of recommendations for Africa by addressing trade, debt, and aid because the G8 Summit still sits high in people's minds. But that's just the beginning. Let me turn to other concrete proposals which strike to the heart of social change, and nothing lies closer to that heart than the plight of women.

I therefore offer a recommendation — the second of the series — that speaks to this most important issue of all. There must be created a true and formidable international agency on behalf of women as part of the multilateral UN system. It can start with a coalition of activist organizations outside the system, and then muscle its way in, but we simply cannot continue to ignore more than half the world's population.

Everyone is in a lather about UN reform, and by the time these lectures are delivered, we will have had the General Assembly debate on the direction of the United Nations over the years ahead. While I cannot predict at this writing what the UN will have done about enlarging the Security Council, or redefining the meaning of terrorism, or reconstituting the Human Rights Commission, or reviewing the international development agenda as embodied in the MDGs, one thing is certain: it will have done nothing to rescue the world's women from the torment of inequality. It won't even have taken the obvious and simple step of demanding an internal UN goal to guarantee a 50/50 split in the employment of women and men at all levels of the United Nations by 2015 (a separate recommendation, and one so overdue that it should be non-negotiable).

And you can be sure that it will have done nothing to address the huge and growing and terrifying vulnerability of the world's women to violence, disease, poverty, and conflict.

That was brought home to me again with a vengeance when I attended, in early June 2005, the United Nations one-day Special Session on HIV/AIDS, whose purpose was to assess the progress that had been made since the Declaration of Commitment on HIV/AIDS at an earlier session in 2001. During the course of the day, I sat through a three-hour "roundtable" on AIDS and gender, during which nineteen governments and a couple of selected NGOs spoke. It was truly dreadful. I've rarely attended a more pointless discussion. The governments were uniformly irrelevant and intellectually vacuous: there was simply the recitation, time and again, of alleged concern about what the pandemic was doing to women, and some vague, rambling responses. A sense of urgency was totally lacking. In fact, in true UN tradition, there was no "discussion" or "roundtable" whatsoever. There was simply a series of prepared solitary statements, relating not at all to any intervention from anyone else.

That's one of the most bizarre things about the United Nations. Everyone religiously sticks to the text drafted in the capitals of their respective countries. If, for example, you were debating a resolution on the banning of nuclear tests, and just as you walked into the conference room it was reported that one hour earlier, North Korea had conducted an underground nuclear explosion, and your text said that the reason for the resolution was the need to prevent further nuclear explosions, you would read your text as though nothing had occurred in the interim.

So it was in the "debate" I endured in June 2005: a series of unrelated remarks, totally shorn of inspiration or application to the real world. You would never know that the lives of the women of the world were at stake. (As a matter of fact, with a certain surrealism, not a single African country took the floor, although there was an intervention — the most intelligent of the day — from the Ethiopian Women Lawyers group.)

I cannot emphasize strongly enough that as part of the reform mandate of the United Nations, the world must come to grips with the need for an overall agency for women. If member states' resistance or budgetary concerns are advanced as excuses to delay its formation, it should be created by activist NGOs outside the UN system and folded in later. But the mind-numbing parade of earnest declarations and reports and unfulfilled Plans of Action must come to an end. I firmly believe a new agency could well be rooted in an amalgamation of the UN Development Fund for Women (UNIFEM), the UN Population Fund (UNFPA), and the Division for the Advancement of Women (DAW) currently placed in the Secretary-General's office. It would have to be headed by an Under-Secretary-General, and funded at no less than the level for UNICEF; that is to say, something close to $2 billion a year.

The difference such an agency would make to Africa alone knows no bounds. At long last, it would be possible for grassroots women leaders to do what they have forever wanted to do — bring together community activists from each and every country in Africa and build a mass women's movement across the continent. The major international conferences of the past two decades have provided abundant proof, if only in teasing glimpses, that every country yields women of vibrant leadership capacity. Were they ever to be given the opportunity on a regular basis to network, plan, share, and plot with their women colleagues in other countries, they could turn the continent on its head. We're talking here about a whole new locus of power — the unleashing of a feminist dynamic to transform Africa, and in the process, rescue women from the cauldron of AIDS. It constitutes a tremendous opportunity for the United Nations to move the sputtering engine of gender equality from neutral into high gear.

I'm advancing this broad proposal for a women's agency in the hope that somewhere, some country, perhaps one of the Nordics, will run with it. I'm proposing it because sometimes at the United Nations, when you hammer home a position time and again, ad nauseam, a modest variation of that position is embraced. I'm proposing it because the situation is desperate beyond desperation. For women, the situation was always desperate, but with the advent of the pandemic, it is as though the lives of women are being held ransom all over the world by the father of all viruses, so virulent, so malevolent as to threaten the very existence of women in some countries, and no one will come to the rescue.

I don't know how often over the last four years I've heard the phrase "women and girls are an endangered species." It's uttered by women's advocates, it's intoned by academic experts, it's used by high-ranking government officials, it's invoked by UN colleagues. Behind the words there lies an inviolable truth: the MDGS are doomed unless we make gender inequality history.

The way in which AIDS exacerbates and accentuates inequality leads me to my next series of proposals for Africa. They are based on the premise of universal treatment for all AIDS patients.

Thus, third, we must maintain the momentum around "three by five," (i.e., the brilliant design by the WHO to put three million people into treatment by the end of this year). We now know that the target will not be reached. It matters not. By the end of this year, we will be verging on one and a half million people in treatment — people who would otherwise be dead. By the time we reach the international AIDS conference in Toronto in August 2006, we'll be very near the three million figure.

It demonstrates that setting goals and targets remains one of the best possible strategies. And in this instance, the proof is in the living.

I remember the derisory and critical comments by Richard Holbrooke, former U.S. ambassador to the United Nations (who played a key role in awakening the UN to the reality of AIDS), attacking the WHO because the target wouldn't be reached. I thought at the time that it set new standards for fatuity. The fact of the matter is that the international community, including the UN, was stagnating in its response to the pandemic until the WHO initiative vaulted upon the scene. "Three by five" has had a remarkable impact: countries are everywhere falling all over themselves to introduce treatment, the numbers are increasing on a daily basis, and hope has re-emerged where only fear and despair held sway.

It was also characteristic of multilateralism that other UN agencies gave the WHO a hard time, and that even within the WHO itself there were grouchy dissidents. There are always internal UN resentments and rivalries that bedevil rational responses (o ye of little minds), and there are always infinite numbers of people who feel that turf and security are threatened by any novel initiative. Worse, there were many people who believed that merely by setting an ambitious target, the WHO was risking credibility and influence.

But the director general of the WHO, Dr. Lee Jong-wook, to his everlasting credit, persevered with resolve and imperturbability. The detractors are routed. The momentum created around "three by five" is now driving everything else, including prevention, which has a new lease on life as a result of treatment. Everywhere, the numbers seeking testing are up, people being far less frightened to know their status. In fact, the time has come to set parallel targets akin to that of treatment, beginning with a goal for voluntary counselling and testing, and another for the prevention of mother-to-child transmission. It is, of course, heartbreaking that treatment is being rolled out so slowly; it is heartbreaking that vast numbers of people will die before treatment is available; it is heart-breaking that we're still dealing with "user fees" for treatment when it should be free; it is heartbreaking that at precisely the moment when treatment is in sight, the pandemic has killed so many health professionals that we lack the human capacity adequately to respond; it is heartbreaking that treatment has been around for nine years in the developed world, and we're only now providing it for Africa.

But this particular breakthrough has finally been made. And the proof of that assertion lies in the language being used. As recently as six months ago, the activist NGOs were thinking about the next arithmetic formulation after "three by five": would it be five by six, seven by seven? No one thinks that way any longer. The NGOs and UNAIDS now uniformly invoke the phrase "universal treatment" or "universal access," understanding that nothing else will be acceptable. Even the G8 felt it necessary to use the words "universal treatment by 2010."

It must bring a smile of vindication to the World Health Organization.

I want to embark on a brief historical excursion at this point, which won't take long, but which has been playing restlessly in my mind, anxious to get out, for three to four years. I had just begun the job of envoy, when I travelled to Rwanda to engage in a number of meetings and field visits. As it happens, it coincided with the World Bank decision to make a large loan to Rwanda under its Multi-country HIV/AIDS Program, known as "MAP," and in a meeting I had with the then World Bank representative in the country, he asked me to support his effort to persuade the Bank headquarters to allow a small percentage of the money to go towards treatment.

I was eager to be of assistance (it may well have been the first time any World Bank official had asked me for a favour; I was probably intoxicated by the whiff of power), and upon returning to Toronto, I phoned a very senior member of the World Bank establishment in Washington who happened to be an admired acquaintance from one of his former incarnations. I laid out the request. I will never, but never forget the gist of the reply (I'm paraphrasing, but paraphrasing with absolute certitude): "You see, Stephen, it's difficult. Let's face the painful truth: the people with AIDS are going to die. The money would probably be better used for prevention. It's all a matter of trade-offs."

I remember nearly jumping through the phone. What World Bank potion had poisoned the progressive leanings of this man whom I liked and respected? I couldn't believe what I was hearing. "Trade-offs," I sputtered. "You speak to me of *trade-offs*? You have drugs to keep people alive, and you're going to let them die because of a trade-off? Why don't you find more money and do both treatment and prevention, and screw the trade-off?"

I lost the argument. But I mention it now because for the longest time, this pernicious frame of mind ruled the dialectical roost. Somehow the people living with AIDS were expendable, in vast numbers, while people in power persuaded themselves that it was better to practise prevention. One of the most excellent things about "three by five" is the way in which it has rejuvenated prevention, and made everyone understand that treatment is far more than treatment, and that treatment and prevention are inseparable.

All of which leads me directly to my fourth proposal: the G8 Summit will inevitably have to confront the shortfall in revenue for the Global Fund to Fight AIDS, Tuberculosis and Malaria. I'm at something of a disadvantage because I'm writing this in the summer of 2005, and the "replenishment conference" for the Global Fund will have been held by the time this lecture is delivered. I can't begin to predict exactly what will happen, but this is unquestionably the critical year for the Global Fund. It requires $700 million more for 2005, $2.9 billion for 2006, and $4.2 billion for 2007, for a total of $7.8 billion. If it doesn't have pledges made for these amounts, it will not be able to review new proposals in 2006 and 2007. Incredibly enough, as things currently stand, the pledges are not in prospect.

It would be an incomparable tragedy if the Global Fund was shortchanged: there is no other international financial vehicle dealing with AIDS that reaches so many people in so many diverse countries, nor any institution so responsive to the demands of the grass-roots. Please note: The Global Fund is operating in 127 countries; it has provided funds to put 200,000 people on antiretroviral treatment, to provide more than 1,000,000 people with voluntary testing and counselling, to put 385,000 on TB treatment, to put 300,000 on malarial treatment, and to provide 1,350,000 families with bed-nets to protect against malaria. In addition, it has reached millions with programs of prevention for all three communicable diseases; it funds training, home-based care, drugs for opportunistic infections, hospital infrastructure, the staffing of National AIDS Councils, and increasingly it provides resources for community-based and faith-based organizations, often working in the world of orphans. There's nothing that approximates the actual and potential scope of the Global Fund.

There's no question that the Global Fund has had growing pains since it came formally into being in 2002. But it has been remarkably adaptive, and has tried vigorously to correct whatever administrative procedures have gone wrong. It is still a work in progress, but a work with great promise and one that is already vital to Africa. It would be a travesty if it failed to receive the money it needs. AIDS, tuberculosis, and malaria collectively take six million lives a year, every year, growing methodically, systematically, relentlessly in number.

The report of the Blair Commission for Africa asserts that the Global Fund must be "fully funded," a good test for the bona fides of the donor world. The most serious obstacle is the United States. The refusal of that country to pull its weight, the offer of a paltry $400 to $600 million for 2006, when the amount should be closer to $1.2 billion, it all amounts to a serious setback for the Global Fund. Again we come back to the G8: how real were the promises? And again it's necessary to emphasize the indispensable advocacy of civil society: holding the feet of the G8 to the Global Fund fire is not just a matter of lobbying, it's a matter of life and death. This is a chance for the NGO community to gain redemption for its passivity at Gleneagles.

But how astonishing is it that even as I write, the NGO community is attempting to mount a campaign to appeal and to beg that the Global Fund experiences no shortfall? We're barely out of the G8 Summit, where promises to help Africa mounted one upon the other like bars of gold at Fort Knox. Does it not say something about the quality of those promises that at the first moment of testing, everyone assumes they will be found wanting?

The summit at Gleneagles was held in the first week of July 2005. The replenishment conference for the Global Fund was held in the first week of September 2005. Anything less than the promise of full funding for 2006 and 2007 mocks the commitments made at Gleneagles. It would appear that it took exactly two months for the inviolable pattern of betrayal of Africa to re-emerge.

It becomes clear in all of this that part of the problem is the almost complete reliance on governments. In my own philosophic view, that reliance is exactly as it should be, except that in the circumstance of AIDS, there is no time for cerebral self-indulgence. The rich countries just won't deliver, and the poor countries can't deliver, and the dying increases exponentially. There have to be alternatives, and I believe they exist.

With the exception of the Gates Foundation, there is no other major AIDS donor from the broadly defined corporate world. This leads me to make a suggestion that the private sector may find perfectly odious, but that I think has some merit.

There is an organization known as the Global Business Coalition on HIV/AIDS, founded and sustained by Richard Holbrooke. Some of the corporate members (many of them multinationals) pursue honourable policies in relation to the pandemic, particularly the provision of medical care, including treatment, for their workers and the workers' families. I've heard presentations from oil companies in Angola and companies like Anglo-American in South Africa that are actually quite moving in their commitment to fighting the pandemic.

What is missing, however, are private sector financial contributions to confront the pandemic on a broader scale, something that would define the true meaning of corporate social responsibility. It should be especially true of those companies that have profited so extravagantly from the resources of the African continent or from the sale of pharmaceuticals. That's not to exempt any others; it's just to identify some obvious candidates.

So here is my proposal: I suggest that all the self-selected members of the Global Business Coalition on HIV/AIDS should contribute 0.7 percent of pre-tax profits to the Global Fund to Fight AIDS, Tuberculosis and Malaria. The target figure is familiar; it has huge international resonance. And there's no reason why, like governments, the corporations shouldn't phase it in between now and 2015 — again in symmetry with international priorities. It would mean a tremendous difference to the Global Fund in its battle against AIDS, and it would make the strongest possible statement, once and for all, that this fight to save humankind is universal.

Fifth, I must attempt to deal with the question of food, which I touched upon in an earlier lecture. A strange thing has been happening internationally which I do not fully understand. There is greater and greater reluctance to provide the funding or the food to feed the hungry, and yet, cutting severe hunger in half by 2015 is, along with a similar reduction in poverty, the first of the MDGS. The most recent example of this perverse state of affairs occurred in Niger in June and July of 2005, when thousands of children actually faced starvation because the international community refused to respond in time to a desperate food shortage.

The executive director of the World Food Programme, James Morris, has made many an eloquent plea for food aid in dollars or in kind for intense human emergencies from Darfur to North Korea to the famine-stricken countries of southern Africa. The response has been lamentable, often less than a quarter of the need. What has gone wrong? Morris is the last person in the world to make requests that could be considered extravagant.

Like replenishing the Global Fund, this, too, is a test of the international community, and a simple one. It might be argued that AIDS is a profoundly complicated subject, wherein every aspect — whether treatment, prevention, or care — involves tortured financial contours on the one hand, and sensitive cultural norms on the other. It can make funding difficult. But hunger is not complicated: starvation is starvation. You don't need a course in human sexuality to grasp the gnawing void of hunger.

As it happens, Morris has understood the force of the pandemic, and is intervening where HIV/AIDS has shredded societies. The WFP is especially supportive of orphan children living in child-headed households; there are many such households that would have no food whatsoever if the WFP was not on the scene. The agency also supports groups of people living with AIDS, actually providing them with food supplements (for most it's not a supplement!) at times of duress. The World Food Programme has grasped the reality of the pandemic's umbilical equation: antiretrovirals don't work on an empty stomach.

Above all, the WFP has become an ever-greater stalwart in the provision of school feeding programs. This is truly excellent. You cannot imagine what it means to children from the most impoverished communities in the world, to be guaranteed one solid meal a day. Inevitably, it's hit and miss — too many impoverished children, too few dollars — but it's hard to find anyone who's associated with school feeding who doesn't feel that it should be universal. At the moment, alas, such thoughts are the stuff of fantasy. The WFP simply doesn't have the money.

As part of the dividing of the spoils from the G8, there must be a new and definitive program for the purchase of food wherever it is needed, or the MDG on hunger is reduced to mere aspiration. But it's much more than that. There must equally be a focus on small agricultural development that dwarfs everything that's gone before. Here, the UN's Food and Agriculture Organization could play a pivotal role, but I get no sense that its upper echelons view things with the sense of emergency that inhabits the WFP. Indeed, I rarely see the UN's Food and Agriculture Organization, FAO, taking leadership on the ground within countries. There was a time, back in the 1980s, while I was at the United Nations for Canada, when the WFP was a sort of branch-plant of the FAO, a mere addendum. If multilateralism were rational rather than self-serving and swamped by vested interests, the countries of the world would fold the FAO into the WFP and see what remarkable improvements might flow for the human condition.

Sixth, there has emerged, because of economist Jeffrey Sachs, one of the more imaginative proposals floating in the ether of social change, the Millennium Village Project. I remember first reading of it in his celebrated new book, *The End of Poverty*, and thinking to myself, "How does he come up with these ideas?" The name Millennium Village Project is entirely apt because Jeffrey is the Special

Advisor to the Secretary-General of the United Nations for the Millennium Development Goals.

The Project conceives of ten villages, of roughly five thousand population each, scattered in various countries throughout Africa. These villages would be given every resource required (primarily dollars, but also expert advice, simple technologies, and infrastructure support) to respond to every human exigency, by rebuilding the interwoven fabric of health care, education, transportation, communications, nutrition, water, sanitation, and, above all, agriculture. I especially appreciate how Jeffrey emphasizes agriculture — every aspect, from soil nutrients to small-scale irrigation — because he understands, as many do not, how agricultural productivity is indispensable to progress on all other fronts.

The decisions on both priorities and implementation will be made at village level, headed by some responsible community leader. It is estimated that the experiment should run for five years at a rough cost of $250,000 to $350,000 annually, or $50 to $70 per person per year (it's amazing, isn't it, how little it takes to resuscitate human lives). In addition, there would be a similar amount devoted to monitoring and evaluating the project as it proceeds, so that impeccable research would be continuously at hand. At this point, there are two villages in process, in Kenya and Ethiopia, with a third in Rwanda just underway. It is all most exciting. I have visited the embryonic village in Kenya, and although one can take issue with this or that aspect, the potential for significant change is indisputable.

The purpose of the exercise is to see if, against all odds, the MDGS can actually be realized at village level with the right kind of financial and technical assistance. The next step is to take it to scale, collaborating with government every step of the way. The bane of Africa's existence at the moment, in response to the pandemic in particular, is the endless number of models, projects, prototypes, and experiments that never get to scale. Many are quite excellent of themselves, but it seems absurd somehow that we never succeed in spreading them across the socio-economic terrain of each of the countries. Success will demonstrate to the world that between daily misery on the one hand, and well-being on the other, there stands only the decision by the rich nations to share a tiny fraction of their wealth.

I suppose I should deal, in passing, with one of the vaguely comical aspects of this subject. People are always asking me how I can consort so closely with Jeffrey Sachs. They even imply a groupie mentality that naturally cuts me to the quick.

Well, let me be absolutely clear. I'm a democratic socialist; my ideology is my life. And it is true to say that Jeffrey Sachs is not a democratic socialist; in fact, although he and I have never discussed it, it would seem from his writings that he's a profoundly misguided democratic capitalist. These are mortal flaws which I charitably overlook. The fact of the matter is, however, that whatever our philosophic differences — and there is no bridge long enough to span the philosophic divide — Jeffrey is quite magnificent in his unswerving pursuit of the end of global poverty, and the amelioration of the human condition. His nostrums may sometimes not be my nostrums. But the power of his intellect and his influence in the service of the most noble of causes are all things I hugely admire, and I'll be damned if I'll allow ideological dogma to get in the way.

We're talking about saving the lives of millions. We're talking about achieving a set of goals never before so fully articulated on behalf of humankind. Jeffrey Sachs is deeply committed to that quest. That's enough for me.

Seventh, there is the question of the "emerging preventive technologies," in particular, vaccines and microbicides. I must admit that in the pantheon of responses to the pandemic, I find the search for a vaccine and the search for a microbicide utterly fascinating. I don't pretend to understand even a snippet of the science, but that's of little consequence.

For me — and this is a personal view based solely on experience, informed by vague dollops of knowledge — at the centre of the hunt for a vaccine is the International AIDS Vaccine Initiative, and the similar role for microbicides is played by the International Partnership for Microbicides.

It has been my good fortune to spend time with both organizations, and to realize what indefatigable effort is going into the discovery of these preventive technologies. A vaccine is obviously the ultimate answer: give us a vaccine, get it out, and the nightmare of millions of new infections winds to an end. However, it would appear, from the opinion of knowledgeable insiders, that a vaccine is ten or more years away. I find that hard to believe, but I'm assured that it is the case. The virus apparently has such capacity for elusive and infinite mutation that no one has yet found the Achilles molecule. Still, I have the absolute conviction that if the greatest-ever research effort was mobilized, surpassing all previous such efforts, dwarfing everything from space shuttles to DNA, we would very soon make the spectacular discovery.

A microbicide, on the other hand, is allegedly not so far off. There are, even now, a number of trials in place at several stages in a number of countries, including African countries, which lead informed people to speculate about a discovery in three to seven years. It is amazing in concept: a microbicide is a cream or gel, which the woman can apply to herself without the partner even knowing, to prevent transmission of the virus. More supernaturally (revealing the extent of my scientific ignorance), there is a product in development which is designed to prevent transmission but permit conception. This would be a tremendous accomplishment, and vital for Africa, where having children is culturally so important.

The crucial factor, in the case of both vaccine and microbicide, is to have access as soon as it is discovered. Thus, advance preparation is underway. It will obviously take significant work, primarily through community health workers, to educate vast numbers of rural women about how to use a microbicide. A vaccine is somewhat easier (immunization is commonplace), but simply fashioning the logistics for distribution will be a great challenge.

Nonetheless, whatever the challenge, we're talking about a lifelong safeguard on the one hand, however far over the horizon, and a way of preventing millions of infections on the other, while the vaccine is awaited. In the early days of infection, it was thought that a vaccine was right around the corner. Today, we're almost a quarter century into the pandemic, and we're still struggling. The issue of resources is also not to be sneezed at: the preventive technologies require a doubling of dollars over the next few years, something in the vicinity of $700 to $800 million more each year. Naturally, the more trials you have in place, the better the prospects for discovery. That takes lots of money, but it's surely a sublime investment.

Eighth, there is the matter of school fees. I've dealt with this, I realize, at some considerable length in an earlier lecture, but I wanted to re-emphasize how crucial it is to devise a plan, country by country, where school fees and every other related cost can be abolished, and where compensatory funding will be available automatically.

My own feeling is that virtually the entire onus should be on the World Bank and the IMF to cough up the money that governments and individual schools lose when the abolition of fees is introduced. After all, the concept of "shared costs" or the equivalent euphemism, "user fees," lies at the root of the destructive fee policy, and those responsible for this ideological *Weltanschauung* should also be responsible for its reversal. This will not be easy. It requires something far more flexible and vastly more imaginative than the so-called "Fast-Track Initiative" administered by the World Bank, which promotes the retrograde notion that donors (most of them utterly ignorant of educational issues) should decide which sovereign developing nations' education plans are worthy of support.

But we're not talking about a privilege to be granted the deserving; we're talking about a fundamental human right that cannot be denied — not to children orphaned by AIDS and not to other vulnerable children, whose need for school is urgent, and whose wherewithal is negligible. Simply put, we're attempting to make real the Millennium Development Goal which says that every child of primary school–going age has the right to be in school.

It is also time, in the pursuit of this objective, to emphasize the very particular role that schools can play in achieving the MDGS. It relates directly to the litany of Quick Wins that were enumerated when the Millennium Development project was issued in document form in January 2005. In addition to fulfilling their traditional roles, schools can also be seen, universally, as natural centres for immunization, deworming, lunch-feeding programs, and the distribution of malarial bed-nets. Add those components to education on HIV/AIDS, the use of the school as a community hub, the school as a water point for the village and a model for a community garden, and you have one of those truly fortuitous combinations that can transform and save a child's life.

Ninth, we come to the question of orphans. As I've moved from country to country over the last four years, it's been clear, inescapably clear, that as the pandemic evolves, children orphaned by AIDS are becoming the single most intractable and painful legacy. There are no equivalent precedents. Nothing in historical experience has prepared us for two generations of children rendered desperate, lonely, sad, and bewildered by sheer circumstance. And it leads to bizarre permutations.

My mind goes back to a recent gathering outside of Kisumu, Kenya, where a community-based organization had assembled a large number of orphan kids to meet with the visiting envoy. In the course of the ceremony (there is always a ceremony), representatives of the orphans were asked to speak, and as they came forward, they turned out, all of them, to be in their early twenties, relating sad and distressing stories about the deaths of their parents several years ago, and the subsequent struggles to keep their families together. The parents had mostly died in the 1990s. That's one of the overlooked and shocking realities about the orphans: the pandemic has been going on so long that the orphans are now adults, and a burgeoning population of parentless children, adolescents, and rootless youth is simply overwhelming for every state. Governments haven't the faintest idea what to do. The policies for orphans, more often than not, are a grab-bag of frantic interventions, where faith-based groups and community-based groups try desperately to cope with the numbers, but rarely have either the capacity or the resources.

The answer to this dire situation lies definitively with UNICEF. In the month of October 2005, the very month when these lectures will be published and delivered, UNICEF is announcing an international plan to raise

$1 billion over six years to respond to the needs of ten million children orphaned by AIDS, or otherwise especially vulnerable. UNICEF has commissioned rapid assessments of the orphan situation in seventeen countries in Africa, and we're told it has potential plans for all. Everyone's hope is that the new executive director of UNICEF, Ann Veneman — a former secretary of agriculture in the Bush cabinet — will take on orphans as the singular *cause célèbre* of her tenure. The orphan predicament is undoubtedly the greatest international challenge that children face.

As part of the nuts and bolts of programming for the orphans, two fascinating dimensions of the response by communities deserve to be included. The first is grandmothers. As I said in my second lecture, grandmothers are assuming the overwhelming burden of care, yet there's almost nothing in the way of special support for the parenting they provide. There's never quite been a sociological phenomenon of this kind: we must collectively carve out a social security scheme for grandmothers, which will permit them to survive themselves, and secure food, clothing, and shelter for their orphan grandchildren.

The second aspect follows logically. The burden of orphans is so horrendous that some countries — Swaziland for sure, with Zambia not far behind — have to establish a whole new cadre of caregivers to look after the children. These caregivers (overwhelmingly women, of course) already assume the maintenance of their own extended families and those of sick and disabled neighbours and friends, and then they're asked to take on even more by virtue of the enveloping tragedy.

In Swaziland, the National AIDS Council came to the conclusion that they needed ten thousand additional caregivers to handle the orphan deluge. There was the most intense debate about whether or not the caregivers should be paid; in Swaziland, as everywhere else in the world, women are expected to engage in voluntary, unacknowledged, and uncompensated caregiving. It was therefore immensely laudable when Swaziland went to the Global Fund and asked for compensation for the ten thousand. Lo and behold, they got it, admittedly only thirty dollars a month, but a significant sum when you consider that people are living on less than a dollar a day.

It's been my hope that the practice would spread to other jurisdictions. And indeed it may. In Swaziland itself, however, the money from the Global Fund has spawned further heated discussion, as the issue became one of equity. What about the thousands of women providing voluntary home-based care to the sick and the dying ("voluntary" being the facile euphemism for women's conscripted labour), who also felt they had a call on payment? What appears to have emerged is a decision to create "pots" of money, in various communities, to which the women will have access as microcredit for income-generating activities. It's not at all the actual payment as originally envisaged, but at least it's a start in the right direction. As everything else where women are concerned, the battle is endless.

In any event, however these things play out, the orphan crisis is, quite simply, monumental. It will get worse. The MDGS on poverty, infant mortality rates, and primary school attendance cannot possibly be reached in the presence of a cataclysm for children of such magnitude.

Allow me, if I may, to add one additional thought. Everyone speaks, with passing ease, about "psycho-social support." That's the term of art. It's meant to convey the therapeutic response to profound emotional distress. In Africa, for children affected by AIDS, except in the rarest of cases, it doesn't exist. I shall never know why we throw it around with such abandon; in fact, it's entirely irresponsible to imply that there's a battalion of social workers and psychologists out there just waiting to intervene. What, for a million orphans? Or would they do group therapy, a thousand at a time? What's more, even if there were some professionals of therapeutic capacity, the individual trauma of loss is so intense that you'd need hours upon hours to plumb the psychic depths of the child and repair the emotional disarray.

What is meant by "psycho-social support" are the sustaining networks of family and friends, which may or may not be adequate. For the child, wrenched from the bosom of the family after a death-watch of months or even years, the informal counselling apparatus leaves much to be desired. There is no question that amongst the responses we must explore is how to handle the psychological lives of children whose emotional equanimity is hanging by a thread. In this world, there are Doctors Without Borders, Engineers Without Borders, there are even Actuaries Without Borders. Of great potential, however, there is an international association of Social Workers Without Borders. If ever they would consider an expanded raison d'être, it should be to rally their potentially multitudinous ranks, and offer to train not only every helping profession in Africa, but legions of community-level paraprofessionals in the art of psychosocial care for orphans.

Tenth, let me say something about human capacity. For as long as I can remember, the term "capacity-building" has been used in the developing world. But in the presence of the pandemic, capacity-building is a palpable misnomer. When so much of your human capacity is dead or ill, it's necessary to talk about capacity replacement or capacity replenishment. Training becomes an imperative part of the process — training of those who are left to be trained, and in the interim, help from abroad to bridge the gap until human capacity is, at least in part, restored. I noticed that everywhere Bill Clinton went, on a pell-mell six-country tour of southern Africa in July 2005, he talked about capacity. No wonder. He was admirably establishing treatment centres for infected children, and in every instance he was forced to bemoan the absence of the professional health workers to provide that treatment. Still, while responding to the pandemic is undoubtedly the most dramatic example of the absence of capacity, each and every one of the MDGS is compromised by a similar deficit.

What is needed, as everyone understands, is a plan, again country by country, sector by sector, to address the shortage. At the moment, no such plan exists, although there are some collaborations between developing and developed country governments, as is the case between Malawi and the United Kingdom. It would also be invaluable to approach this and similar problems through unusual regional groupings, possibly organized on the basis of highest prevalence rates (Botswana, Swaziland, Lesotho, Namibia, Zimbabwe), or greatest numbers of people infected (South Africa, India, Nigeria, Ethiopia), or best drug procurement strategies (Zambia, Rwanda, Brazil, Thailand).

Coordinated leadership is what's missing from any plans to deal with capacity, and I can't but believe that the leadership should come from the United Nations. Not the money, not the person power, not even the plans themselves, but most emphatically the leadership to get the job done. The UN has all of the country presence imaginable; the UN country teams are the obvious resource to take the lead.

Finally, as I gradually wind my way to the end of these lectures, I want to raise what I would call "matters of controversy." For reasons that will become self-evident, this is not going to be easy for me. But I believe it must be done.

My experience of the last twenty years in the multilateral system has been an absorbing lesson in the wiles and arts of diplomacy. One learns, sometimes through painful experience, that as a UN bureaucrat, it's not always possible to criticize individual countries without arousing occasional bouts of indignation and anger, not to mention threats of retaliation. In my own view, multilateralists are far too often guilty of self-censorship, but there is a price to be paid for candour.

On two occasions, I was forced to beat a partial retreat after boldly naming names. The first involved China, whose policy of incarcerating disabled children in filthy and punitive orphanages I attacked on the basis of a superb monograph published by Human Rights Watch. I was deputy executive director of UNICEF at the time. Members of the Chinese Mission to the United Nations marched into my office in a diplomatic lather. We arrived at a satisfying compromise which involved UNICEF monitoring the orphanages and training the staff, but not before I tendered a strangled apology. The second instance — also during my days as deputy — involved Sudan, and a successful coup by UNICEF in managing to rescue fourteen abducted Ugandan children. They had been held captive in Sudan by a lunatic, vaguely religious group called the Lord's Resistance Army, operating from military camps on Sudanese soil with the full knowledge of the Sudanese government. In this instance a formal complaint was registered by the government of Sudan, although UNICEF retreated not one inch. But I had to be excessively careful: the Sudanese government, which detested me with near-venom, issued veiled threats against UNICEF personnel in Sudan. I was, after all, safely in New York.

I've often been sobered when thinking of those experiences, and the travails of other colleagues in analogous circumstances. But all of that caution is thrown to the wind in the presence of the pandemic. I am personally persuaded that the toll on society from AIDS, the threat to the very underpinnings of African survival is so intense, that the normal diplomatic proprieties must be abandoned. I would argue that it's morally irresponsible to embrace silence when there's so much at stake. I must admit that I'm emboldened in part because of the changing international atmosphere: after all, we're now talking about the "right to protect" (a particularly Canadian construct), which suggests the international right to intervene in situations where nation states are not upholding the human rights of their citizens, Darfur being the most dramatic current example. If the "right to protect" had existed at the time of Rwanda, there might not have been a genocide.

Does that logic apply to AIDS? Not in a symmetrical way, I guess. You couldn't march a UN force into a country because the country refused to take HIV/AIDS seriously. But I think the growing international impatience with the behaviour of some nation states suggests that at least we can be more forthright, without counselling extreme measures. And being more forthright can achieve a great deal.

I think that the pandemic of HIV/AIDS forces us, all of us, to speak out when we think transgressions are being committed. If Colin Powell was right when he was secretary of state — as I believe he was — to say that AIDS was the most significant threat in the world, greater even than weapons of mass destruction, then I believe that the assertion of principle must replace the reliance on niceties.

For example, the U.S. President's Emergency Plan for AIDS Relief, or PEPFAR, as it's colloquially known, cannot escape criticism simply because it's so potentially potent in scope, or because it comes from the world's superpower. When PEPFAR was first announced, everyone was predictably stunned at the amount of money: $15 billion over five years. It eclipsed by far anything undertaken by former President Clinton. And everyone was initially willing to give PEPFAR the benefit of the doubt. Even I — unrepentant social democrat, unrepentant critic of the Bush regime — recognized that the sums were so large they couldn't but do some good. On those grounds alone, along with so many others, I initially suspended negative comment.

And the Bush initiative has done a great deal of good. I'm not so foolhardy as to deny it. You pump that much money, in increments, into a sick and ailing health-care system, and significant numbers of people will benefit in ways large and small, including from life-saving treatment.

But that's not really the critical point. The point is the significant numbers who might have benefited and have been excluded; the point is the conditions that have been imposed by the administration which are unnecessarily destructive.

The choice of countries leaves much to be desired. Swaziland, with the highest prevalence rate in the world, is excluded. Lesotho, with the highest prevalence rate amongst the least developed countries, is excluded. Malawi, with the most abject situation of human capacity this side of Afghanistan, is excluded. The Americans will argue that there's the Millennium Challenge Account which will service the needs of those countries, but so far, as indicated earlier, that account has rendered only paltry proceeds.

PEPFAR is subject to skepticism on several other grounds as well. The amount of money going to the Global Fund is grossly inadequate. There's just no comparison between the two: the Global Fund is in scores and scores of countries; PEPFAR is in fifteen. If this were a world where ideology was not so extreme, and the anti-multilateral impulse in the United States were not so strong, all of the money would have gone to the Global Fund, and great things would have been accomplished. As it is, thus far only $300 million to $500 million a year has been allocated to the Global Fund, representing between 10 to 16 percent of the annual $3 billion total which the United States has available. Sad, very sad.

And then there's the purchase, so far exclusively, of brand-name drugs, at prices far in excess of generic AIDS drugs. The argument is that the United States would not distribute drugs in developing countries that have not been approved by the U.S. Food and Drug Administration (FDA). This seemingly principled position has the useful side effect of pumping American dollars into the coffers of brand-name U.S. drug manufacturers. Even if, under public pressure (and the pressure has been intense), some generics are approved by the FDA, you can be sure that the balance sheets of the brand-name pharmaceutical industry will somehow remain buoyant.

Let it be noted that the present set of generics now used in developing countries are approved, or "prequalified," by the WHO, based on the work of international scientists whose expertise rivals that of any others in the world. Generic "fixed-dose combinations" — three antiretroviral drugs in one capsule or pill — are now used to treat hundreds of thousands of people throughout the world with great effect, and they are distributed by a splendid consortium of purchasers made up of the Clinton Foundation, the World Bank, the Global Fund, and UNICEF. Case closed.

Well, perhaps not quite so quickly. There is also the U.S. policy, applied specifically to PEPFAR funds, requiring a focus on abstinence rather than condoms. Pitting one against the other is abundantly absurd, but the policy as policy is untenable: just how, for example, does a married woman protect herself when she can't practise abstinence and she suspects her husband isn't faithful, and what happens to young people who do not accept the American imprimatur that abstinence is best, but choose instead to be sexually active?

No one in my acquaintance, involved seriously in fighting the pandemic, diminishes the value of abstinence, but no such person would contemplate for a moment casting aspersions on condoms, the most effective preventive method of them all. In a similar context is the recent U.S. policy requiring all NGO recipients of foreign aid dollars to sign an agreement that they will not support prostitution. This ideological (read: fundamentalist) fiat has the effect of compromising projects involving commercial sex workers, who are obviously key to fighting the pandemic. Brazil, with perhaps the best prevention policies in the world, has refused a grant of $40 million from the United States, rather than submit to any such irrational (and odious) requirement. No one promotes prostitution, but it's counter-productive to dismiss and isolate a group that is so important in the fight against the pandemic.

It would seem that over time, PEPFAR and various governments, plus the Global Fund, are getting along better, subduing the tensions, and finding a basis for co-operation. That's all to the good. But we have lost a tremendous opportunity to break the back of the pandemic, and we should not be afraid to say so, simply because of the intimidation of strength and power.

However, let me shift grounds if I may. There's also the case of recalcitrant African countries which must be faced. This is a vastly more difficult proposition.

What, for example, does one do about Zimbabwe? It's rather a double whammy. On the one hand, Zimbabwe is the perfect example of making the people of a country suffer mightily because donor governments dislike the leader, Robert Mugabe, and refuse, therefore, to transfer resources. On the other hand, Zimbabwe is an example of a country where the indices of health and poverty are in a downward spiral, in significant part because of the policies of the government. Figures recently released by UNICEF showing the incalculable damage to children are truly shocking.

The pandemic is particularly gruesome in Zimbabwe, and though President Mugabe has begun to speak out, the toll in a country with a prevalence rate of 25 percent seems to know no bounds. It becomes necessary, I think, for people in authority at the United Nations to convey to the president and his colleagues that the levels of internal destabilization are making an adequate response to AIDS impossible. It is not tolerable that the risk of the virus should be compounded by political turbulence. One of the ugliest episodes of 2005 was the slum-razing in Zimbabwe, instituted by Mugabe, resulting not only in massive human displacement, but disrupting treatment and literally jeopardizing life for large numbers of people living with AIDS. The Secretary-General's appointment of the executive director of UN-Habitat, Anna Tibaijuka, to investigate the ruthless slum clearance in Zimbabwe and issue a report (a report which resulted in explicit condemnation) is an example of the kind of initiative that the United Nations should regularly be taking.

In a similar vein, an arrangement must be bartered among the donor community, the NGOs, and the government to allow the pandemic to be addressed as it is being addressed in the surrounding countries. The WFP has managed to keep the doors open with the regime. It's not always an easy relationship, but the WFP is impressive in the arrangements made to keep people fed. Perhaps they should broker the entente on AIDS. Someone has to do it; the United Nations is best placed. We've all prevaricated for far too long.

And what does one do about Swaziland? Here we have a king who defiantly practises polygamy, who takes more than a dozen wives, the most recent but sixteen years of age, who talks of building them individual palaces, and sweeps across the Swaziland stage in new-fangled cars of outrageous price.

In the meantime, his "subjects" are dying in numbers that would have made Malthus weep, living in a country with the highest prevalence rate in the world — the most recent estimate, based on antenatal sites, having risen to 42 percent! And all of us are quiet; nary an audible peep from the UN family.

How is this silence anything other than complicity? As I said before, I'm not suggesting that the "right to protect" is the right to intervene, but surely it is the right to denounce. Believe me, I know how tough it is. When I visited Swaziland, I met at length with the king in private, and attempted to persuade him, with a combination of subtlety and argument, that the world was increasingly impatient, his people were decimated, and his behaviour was unacceptable. Then we held a press conference together and I held my tongue.

I have felt guilty about that to this day. Whom did it serve but the bloated ego of the monarch? So I've rationalized my actions: I've persuaded myself that it's not for me to do, that it should be done by UN officials with far greater authority. I'm merely a part-time envoy.

But I know my excuses for remaining silent in the face of such behaviour don't wash. And I don't understand why my UN colleagues are prepared to put up with the behaviour. This is one instance where the country is sufficiently small and sufficiently vulnerable to feel compelled to take its critics seriously. Even the king would be forced to take notice.

Look at what our silence hides: Polygamy, which denigrates women and spreads the virus; early marriage, which directly violates UN conventions (ratified by Swaziland!); monumental extravagance in the face of pernicious illness and misery. It's alright to speak out about Darfur, about the Congo, about northern Uganda, but not about Swaziland? Conflict is indictable, but wanton death from disease is acceptable?

And what about the toughest of them all: South Africa? Let me bare my soul, even though I may be courting trouble. But then again, even though I have a specific role as UN envoy, I'm a Canadian, speaking in my own country, delivering the Massey lectures. I'm putting the self-imposed muzzle aside.

Every senior UN official, engaged directly or indirectly in the struggle against AIDS, to whom I have spoken about South Africa, is completely bewildered by the policies of President Mbeki. That is not a revelation, I'm sure. What is true, I believe, of all of us, is a tremendous commitment to South Africa — a confidence that South Africa is the centrepiece of the continent, and that we would do anything and everything in our power to support its growth and development. Many of us were in some way involved in the international battle against apartheid: not a one of us didn't weep when Nelson Mandela took his long walk to freedom.

But something has gone wrong with the post-Mandela government. I have expressed concerns about the government's economic policies on other occasions, but I shall not do so now because it's not the focus of this lecture. I am, however, deeply concerned by the slow rollout of treatment for those living with the AIDS virus in South Africa — and now we know, as a result of the most recent report from the Ministry of Health, that there are well over six million people infected, the highest absolute number of infections in the world. I would have thought that the latest figures would strike the fear of the Almighty into the heart of the government; that they would accelerate the rollout of treatment as though there were no tomorrow, because without treatment, there *is* no tomorrow.

On matters of budgetary allocation, on matters of prevention and care, the government is doing some excellent things. But on treatment it is lagging unconscionably, and too many people are dying to allow for the lag.

Unfathomable comments by the minister of health don't help matters. She perpetually and publicly advocates nutritional remedies for a deadly disease. If she feels garlic and sweet potatoes are indispensable to maintain the health of HIV-positive people, then so be it. But it's going too far to let garlic and sweet potatoes appear to equal or transcend antiretroviral treatment in importance, nor should wantonly exaggerated rumours about the side effects of treatment be allowed to stir confusion in the public. This is not an admirable stance. If my colleagues and friends are confused by the position of the president, they are incredulous at the words and actions of the minister of health.

Over the last four years, I have been to every country in East and southern Africa, many of them two, three, and four times. I can say, confidently and categorically, that every single country (with the exception of newly peaceful Angola, whose borders were closed to traffic — and the virus — throughout the civil war) is working harder at treatment than is South Africa, with fewer relative resources, and in most cases nowhere near the infrastructure or human capacity of South Africa. It is a situation which is absolutely mystifying.

What troubles me, and troubles me deeply, is that the United Nations knows that something is terribly wrong, and yet we feel we can't say anything about it. Even as I write, I'm being consciously guarded. The only senior UN official who has spoken out is Dr. Jim Kim, head of HIV/AIDS at the WHO, who has had the courage to say that one of the reasons we won't make the overall "three by five" treatment target is the slowness of the South African rollout.

I hope with all my heart that things change between the time of this writing and the time of publication. But I won't hold my breath. I don't know how magnificent organizations like the Treatment Action Campaign in South Africa, working on behalf of millions of people living with the virus, manage to maintain their cool as their members and supporters die by the thousands every week. For them, it feels like crimes against humanity.

The mood swings around HIV/AIDS are fascinating. The same experts and commentators, in any given brief period, can ricochet from hope to desolation. At one moment, we're ahead of the pandemic; the next moment, we're behind the pandemic. I've often given messages so mixed that listeners must wonder, wherein lies the truth? But the truth is that truth inhabits both ends of the spectrum. At the level of the grand design — more money, more drugs, more prevention, more care — hope is instinctive. On the ground, where people live and die, where the grand design has yet to be felt, the pandemic is hell on earth.

You can't avoid its cruelty. Not long ago, I visited a little unincorporated town on the outskirts of Lusaka, Zambia. The citizens of the township proudly showed me their graded road and a cinder-block community centre which served, as well, as a local school. Then they asked me to say a few words of appreciation.

We gathered on the gravelly knoll outside the community centre, several hundred strong. And as I was surveying the crowd, just about to speak, I suddenly realized something that jolted me to my inner being. In the front row was a group of very young mothers — mostly in their older teens or perhaps in their early twenties — with their infant babes at their breasts, and everyone else, except for children, was elderly. I could scarce credit it. There were hardly any people in their later twenties, thirties, forties, or fifties. I asked the crowd how many were grandparents, and the majority of hands shot up. I asked how many were looking after orphan grandchildren, and a majority of hands shot up.

There it was, visually: the new face of large parts of Africa. Or perhaps one should say, the absent face of Africa.

My own view is that the horrendous toll is yet to come. Countries will be fighting for survival ten and fifteen years down the road. It's simply impossible to tear the productive generations out of the heart of a country without facing an incomparable crisis. When people say, sometimes triumphantly, that prevalence rates have levelled off, what they mean most often is that the number of people who have died equals the number of new infections. It's *mathematicus diabolus*.

I live in hope. After all, if the Millennium Development Goals are not to be a mockery, then the virus will have to be subdued. Maybe the MDGs will provide the impetus that's needed on AIDS.

But I also live in rage. I've told audiences before, and I'll say it again: I'm not some sweet innocent; I'm sixty-seven years old; I've learned something about politics, diplomacy, and multilateralism. I thought I understood the way the world works. I don't. I'll devote every fibre of my body to defeating this viral contagion, but I cannot abide the wilful inattention of so much of the international community. I cannot expunge from my mind the heartless indifference, the criminal neglect of the last decade, during which time countless people have gone to their graves — people who should still be walking the open savannah of Africa.

In 2005, the world will pass the trillion-dollar mark in the expenditure, annually, on arms. We're fighting for $50 billion annually for foreign aid for Africa: the military total outstrips human need by 20 to 1. Can someone please explain to me our contemporary balance of values?

GLOSSARY

ADF	African Development Forum
antiretrovirals	drugs for the treatment of AIDS
the Bank	World Bank
Beijing	Fourth World Conference on Women, held in Beijing, China, in 1995
Blair Commission	expert working group on aid to Africa commissioned by U.K. Prime Minister Tony Blair, authors of the March 11, 2005, report "Our Common Interest"
Bono	rock star and co-founder of the non-profit organization Debt AIDS Trade Africa (DATA)

Cairo	International Conference on Population and Development, held in Cairo, Egypt, in 1994
CBC	Canadian Broadcasting Corporation
CD4 count	a measure of the body's infection-fighting white blood cells, used to determine when AIDS treatment should begin
CEDAW	Convention on the Elimination of All Forms of Discrimination Against Women
CIA	United States Central Intelligence Agency
CIDA	Canadian International Development Agency
Commission for Africa	see above: "Blair Commission" report
Dakar	World Education Forum, held in Dakar, Senegal, in 2000
DAW	United Nations Division for the Advancement of Women

Doha round	the set of World Trade Organization negotiations that began in Doha, Qatar, in 2001
FAO	United Nations Food and Agriculture Organization
FDA	United States Food and Drug Administration
FTI	Fast-Track Initiative, a World Bank–administered process for identifying the developing country education plans that are considered suitable for donors' support
the Fund	International Monetary Fund
G7	the name now given to meetings of the finance ministers of seven of the "Group of Eight" (see "G8" below)
G8	the "Group of Eight," a grouping of seven of the world's leading industrialized, democratic nations (Canada, France, Germany, Italy, Japan, the United Kingdom, and the United States), plus Russia

Geldof	Bob Geldof, musician and organizer of the 1985 "Live Aid" benefit concert for Ethiopia, and the 2005 "Live 8" concerts to call attention to global poverty
generics	unbranded versions of brand-name medications
Gleneagles	the July 2005 G8 Summit held in Gleneagles, Scotland
the Global Fund	the Global Fund to Fight AIDS, Tuberculosis and Malaria
IFIS	the International Financial Institutions, including the World Bank, the International Monetary Fund, the African Development Bank, and other regional development banks
ILO	United Nations International Labour Organization
IMF	International Monetary Fund
Jo'burg	Johannesburg, South Africa
Jubilee 2000	global movement to cancel the international debts owed by impoverished countries

Live 8	a series of rock concerts in July 2005 staged in eight major cities to call attention to global poverty and influence world leaders attending the G8 Summit meeting
London Club	informal group of commercial banks that join together to negotiate their claims against a sovereign debtor*
Madiba	colloquial name of Nelson Mandela
Make Poverty History	global movement on behalf of developing countries that promotes trade justice, debt cancellation, more and better aid, and full funding to address HIV/AIDS
MAP	World Bank's Multi-country HIV/AIDS Program for Africa
MDGS	Millennium Development Goals
Monterrey	Financing for Development Conference held in Monterrey, Mexico, in 2002
MSF	Médecins Sans Frontières (Doctors Without Borders)

* From the IMF website

NDP	New Democratic Party of Canada
nevirapine	drug prescribed for HIV and AIDS patients, and to prevent the transmission of HIV during labour and delivery
NGO	non-governmental organization
ODA	Official Development Assistance
Paris Club	informal group of official creditors, mostly industrialized countries, that discusses financial arrangements for debtor nations
PEPFAR	U.S. President's Emergency Plan For AIDS Relief
PLWA	People Living With AIDS
PMTCT	Prevention of Mother-to-Child Transmission
PMTCT-*Plus*	Prevention of Mother-to-Child Transmission along with AIDS treatment for the mother, her partner, and family
SAP	Structural Adjustment Program

three by five	United Nations initiative to put 3 million people with HIV/AIDS into antiretroviral treatment in developing countries by the end of 2005
UNAIDS	Joint United Nations Programme on HIV/AIDS
sibling families	children living alone after the deaths of their parents
UNDP	United Nations Development Programme
UNESCO	United Nations Educational, Scientific and Cultural Organization
UNFPA	United Nations Population Fund
UNICEF	United Nations Children's Fund
UNIFEM	United Nations Development Fund for Women
universal treatment	antiretroviral therapy for everyone who requires it
Uruguay round	the series of World Trade Organization negotiations that began in Uruguay and lasted from 1986 to 1994

VCT	voluntary and confidential counselling and testing for HIV/AIDS
WFP	United Nations World Food Programme
WHO	World Health Organization

The CBC Massey Lectures Series

Race Against Time
Stephen Lewis
0-88784-733-1 (p)

A Short History of Progress
Ronald Wright
0-88784-706-4 (p)

The Truth About Stories
Thomas King
0-88784-696-3 (p)

Beyond Fate
Margaret Visser
0-88784-679-3 (p)

The Cult of Efficiency
Janice Gross Stein
0-88784-678-5 (p)

The Rights Revolution
Michael Ignatieff
0-88784-656-4 (p)

The Triumph of Narrative
Robert Fulford
0-88784-645-9 (p)

Becoming Human
Jean Vanier
0-88784-631-9 (p)

The Elsewhere Community
Hugh Kenner
0-88784-607-6 (p)

The Unconscious Civilization
John Ralston Saul
0-88784-586-x (p)

On the Eve of the Millennium
Conor Cruise O'Brien
0-88784-559-2 (p)

Democracy on Trial
Jean Bethke Elshtain
0-88784-545-2 (p)

Twenty-First Century Capitalism
Robert Heilbroner
0-88784-534-7 (p)

The Malaise of Modernity
Charles Taylor
0-88784-520-7 (p)

Biology as Ideology
R. C. Lewontin
0-88784-518-5 (p)

The Real World of Technology
Ursula Franklin
0-88784-636-x (p)

Necessary Illusions
Noam Chomsky
0-88784-574-6 (p)

Compassion and Solidarity
Gregory Baum
0-88784-532-0 (p)

Prisons We Choose to Live Inside
Doris Lessing
0-88784-521-5 (p)

Latin America
Carlos Fuentes
0-88784-665-3 (p)

Nostalgia for the Absolute
George Steiner
0-88784-594-0 (p)

Designing Freedom
Stafford Beer
0-88784-547-9 (p)

The Politics of the Family
R. D. Laing
0-88784-546-0 (p)

The Real World of Democracy
C. B. Macpherson
0-88784-530-4 (p)

The Educated Imagination
Northrop Frye
0-88784-598-3 (p)